MW01234215

PRAISE for Making the SHiFT®

"No yoga or therapy session can compare. If you want relief and success in your life, you must SHiFT® immediately. You are worth it."

- Dorothy Breininger, Expert, *Hoarders* TV Show, Founder of Boss Organizer Blueprint

"SHiFT®, a method to organize developed by Jen Cazares, is a unique and timely program to embrace. When people talk about getting organized, they imply that it's a one-and-done operation. This is just not true. Being organized is a way to live your life and impacts every aspect of your life. Through her SHiFT® approach to organizing, Jen teaches people how to alter their interactions with stuff so they can truly live the life they deserve."

- Diane N. Quintana, Master Trainer, CPO-CD®, CPO®, DNQ Solutions, LLC, Release, Repurpose, Reorganize, LLC

"I love the practical advice and client stories. Jen brings the organizing work she does to life!"

- Laurene Livesey-Park, CPO-CD®, Certification and Services Director, Institute for Challenging Disorganization® (ICD®)

"'E' is for 'Essential!' This book is a must for anyone assisting those challenged by disorganization in their home, space, and life. The author, who is an experienced and compassionate professional organizer, addresses the many roadblocks—including one's own mindset—that a person may encounter while trying to get organized. Her holistic and comprehensive approach provides an easy-to-follow method to forming new, sustainable organizing habits."

- Jill B. Yesko, Certified Professional Organizer and Author of *I'm Right Here: 10 Ways to Get Help for Chronic Disorganization* and *Chronological Order: The Fine Print for a Large Life*

"*Making the SHiFT®* will inspire and provide hope to those experiencing severe disorganization in their lives. Jen founded the acronym SHiFT® to emphasize the five main intangible elements that are frequently overlooked. Using the SHiFT® approach during the organizing process, where one can examine those psychological intangibles, is brilliant. Her client experiences and perspectives provide a helpful tool for tackling a complex topic and offers clutter liberation, restored dignity, and joy for all those in need."

- Sheila S. Delson, CPO-CD®, ICD® Master Trainer, CVOP™

MAKING THE

SHiFT®

True Stories of How People Affected by
Chronic Disorganization Learn to Live a Deserving Life

Jen Cazares, CPO-CD®, CVOP™

with contributor Connie Anderson, CPO-CD®

Foreword by Judith Kolberg

Published by Livable Spaces®, LLC

Book cover design by Beckie Reay ©NorthRose Studio

Interior design by Ian White www.ianpauljameswhite.com

"Should I Try Virtual Organizing?" chart by Hazel Thornton

ISBN: 979-8-218-09341-9

Printed in the United States of America

Requests for bulk orders, permission to make copies of any part of this book, or other inquiries can be made by contacting:

Livable Spaces®, LLC
(925) 367-8300
jen@livablespaces.net
LivableSpaces.net

DEDICATION

To my client Don, one of the kindest, most generous people I have known. You gave this struggle your all, and I will admire you forever for that. We hugged, and you shed a tear of relief and hope, saying to me, "Don't ever leave me, Jen." I said back, "Don, I will never leave you." I know your life on earth was a difficult one and far too short, but I know you are in a compassionate, loving place now.

DISCLAIMERS

First, while SHiFT® addresses topics such as mental health, physical health, and finances, neither I nor my contributor Connie Anderson is an expert in those fields. We don't claim to be psychologists, medical professionals, or Certified Financial Planners. What we *can* do is offer guidance to you and your clients to set up systems related to these areas in your clients' lives. For example, I don't prescribe a specific nutrition plan, but I can help you and your client create a kitchen that supports a healthy lifestyle. Connie and I encourage you to seek advice from other professionals for issues that are outside the scope of this book.

Second, to protect and honor the identities of the clients we work with, Connie and I have altered their names and omitted details that would identify them. We made a pledge to them to be nonjudgmental and confidential. The circumstances and environments recounted in these chapters are true. They reflect both unique situations and common qualities found in the chronic disorganization community, which we hope will be instructive.

TABLE OF CONTENTS

FOREWORD

by Judith Kolberg

*Founder of the Field of Professional Organizing That
Serves Individuals with Chronic Disorganization*

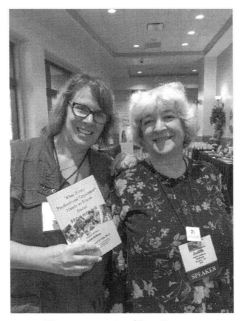

Photo property of Jen Cazares

***Jen, holding one of Judith's books in 2017—the
year Jen began her journey to become a CPO-CD®***

Chronic disorganization (CD) is hard to address. It takes the
on-the-ground effort of a skillful team; an active collaboration
between client, professional organizer, and other professionals;
and a high-level understanding of the specific effect of CD on

a person's unique life. *Making the SHiFT®, True Stories of How People Affected by Chronic Disorganization Learn to Live a Deserving Life* is a bold book that integrates the problems a person with CD exhibits into solutions uniquely crafted for them. Captured in the clever acronym SHiFT®, the methodology examines "S," the impact of CD on a person's capacity to form and enjoy a social life. It looks at "H," the physical and mental health of their client. It uses "I" to represent "I am deserving," the professional commitment to respecting and honoring every individual's self-worth. It recognizes that CD typically strains "F," a person's finances, with debt, excessive shopping, and lack of money management. And finally, SHiFT® explores "T," for time management, a skill most CD people lack.

It is not easy to convert the intimate lived experience of working side-by-side with a CD client into concrete exercises. Yet Jennifer Cazares approaches this task bravely through a series of self-awareness tools like the Thought Box and the Think, Write...Deserve exercise. But the heart of this book is the true stories Cazares tells of clients who begin hopeless and, by working through the SHiFT® Method, learn to live happy, deserving, organized lives. These stories are full of empathy, support, and hope. In my opinion, there can never be enough empathy, support, and hope for CD folks.

INTRODUCTION

Becoming a Professional Organizer

"The more you know why you do the things you do and the more purpose you feel in every step, the more likely it is you can improve the world as a whole, too."

—MasterClass

I did not grow up imagining I would one day write, and certainly not a book for fellow professional organizers. In fact, until several years ago, I had never heard of professional organizing. Isn't everyone naturally organized? Why would you need someone to teach you how to get organized?

I grew up in rural Northern California, where I hunted, fished, and foraged. Growing up in the country requires some level of self-sufficiency, but my brother and I also had to learn these skills because our parents weren't always available. While my mom was affectionate, generous, and outwardly loving on her good days, she had many depressive episodes throughout my childhood. Meanwhile, my dad was aloof and often drank too much. As a result, my parents argued a lot. To cope with their arguments, I took comfort in food. It became my go-to escape from the tension and stress in the household.

My literal escape came when I had the chance to attend boarding school for high school. From there, I went off to college, where I earned a double degree in Business Administration and English. Little did I know the classes I took in psychology would turn out to be the most useful years later, when I began my organizing career.

After college, I worked in human resources for a major fashion retail company and then for a car dealership. I loved training employees, and I made myself available to them both inside my human resources role and on the car dealership sales floor. I found that I could relate to their issues of being overworked, underpaid, and generally taken advantage of by the company. These were issues I wanted to help them fix. I did my best, but it was an uphill battle. Eventually, I left the corporate world to start a catering business. I was tired of seeing people struggle against the system, and I was ready to be my own boss.

During this time of professional exploration, I got married. Unfortunately, from the day we said "I do," I knew my first husband was not right for me. Yet I ignored that inner voice and allowed life to move forward—which had consequences. Being around his family while harboring doubts about our relationship caused me so much stress that one month after our wedding, I had a stroke. I was only twenty-nine. Over the next several months of medical appointments, I experienced more neurological problems, migraines, and balance issues. Finally, my medical team performed a spinal tap and diagnosed me with multiple sclerosis.

While this news was terrifying, in a way it also freed me. I left my loveless marriage and eventually found a new partner, who is now the love of my life. I also started to work my way out of the depths of depression, which I had attempted to self-treat with 125 extra pounds of bodyweight "protection." Finally, with the help of a therapist and a whole lot of work, I was beginning to see the light at the end of the tunnel.

Several years later, through my son's school's PTA, I had a chance encounter with Connie Anderson—the first of many professional organizers I would eventually meet. It was fortuitous timing, because I was at a professional crossroads: I wanted to leave the catering business, but I couldn't stomach the idea of going back to the corporate world. As we became friendly, Connie told me about her profession. When I expressed interest, she connected me with another organizer who was willing to take me along so I could see what it was all about. This organizer was working in a hoarded home, which she told me was a Level III on the Clutter–Hoarding Scale®. At the time,

I didn't know anything about the Clutter–Hoarding Scale®, but I thought, "What the hell, I'll do it!" When I saw the hoarded house we were about to tackle, my mind was blown. "People live like this? And other people are paid to help them?"

As I teamed up with Connie on more and more jobs, my fascination with the industry grew. She told me about the Institute for Challenging Disorganization® and officially introduced me to the Clutter–Hoarding Scale®. I soon learned the meaning of hoarding disorder and what it meant when Connie called a client a "Level III." Three years later, I earned my certification as a Certified Professional Organizer in Chronic Disorganization® (CPO-CD®). The work I've been doing since has been some of the most gratifying work I've ever done. I am making a real difference in people's lives.

The paradox of my life is that all of the challenges that seem to have left me broken—my upbringing, my toxic marriage, my multiple sclerosis diagnosis—have made me more compassionate and empathetic to other people's struggles, especially those with the most severe cases of CD. I wonder if they feel unworthy of a comfortable home. Is their sense of self-worth and self-esteem so weak that they just stopped trying to care for themselves? At one time or another, I also felt hopeless, helpless, and overwhelmed. My clients' stuff provides them with the same protection and comfort as food once did for me. My extra pounds made me feel safe, just like the clutter makes them feel safe—whether they're aware of it or not. This layer of protection fills a void where love, acceptance, and belonging are missing. I may never have lived in a house overwhelmed by clutter, but I have absolutely experienced the internal void my clients feel and the sense of worthlessness that comes with it. I am committed to helping these individuals find the self-love and worthiness that they deserve.

As I write this book, my multiple sclerosis has progressed. Currently, I am struggling with the physical demands of organizing people's stuff, and I anticipate that my day-to-day on-site organizing work with clients will taper off. That is, in large part, why I've written this book. My clients and I have had immense success with the SHiFT® Method. This method goes beyond the surface-level "cleaning and tidying" that happens so often when individuals with CD try to get organized and taps into the root of the problem. That is, it not only helps individuals get organized but shifts their whole mindset and their view of themselves.

My goal is to make my own successes the successes of every professional organizer. I've seen this method give people with CD and their families hope. With practice, we have seen real, lasting results. By the end of the book, my promise is that you will have the tools you need to bring those same results to your clients. You will be ready to give those challenged by CD the hope and the change they need to live full, deserving lives.

Chapter 1

Identifying Chronic Disorganization

"Ability is what you're capable of doing. Motivation determines what you do. Attitude dictates how well you do it."

—unknown

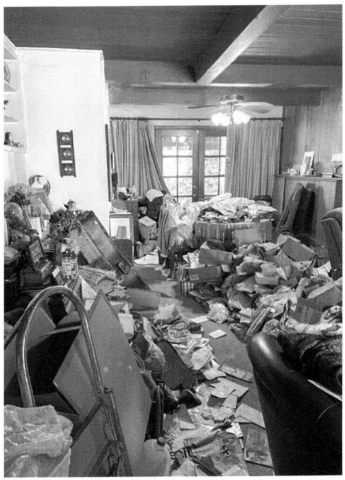

Photo credit: Jen Cazares

A hoarded house reflects what's going on in the mind of someone with CD: internal chaos.

There are hundreds, possibly even thousands, of books on "how to get organized." Some send you to The Container Store, others use a ranking system, and still others offer mindfulness tactics and list-making strategies. These methods work well for folks trying to tackle ordinary issues around disorganization. After all, we've all forgotten our cell phone on the way out the door, punched in late for work, or spent thirty minutes trying to find a tax form from two years ago. That's life! And a little self-help can go a long way toward preventing those inconveniences.

The problem is when the inconveniences become constant. If they're happening nearly every day, to the point where they're impacting a person's living space and ability to function, the root issue might be something more than run-of-the-mill disorganization. It might be chronic disorganization.

What Is Chronic Disorganization?

According to the Institute for Challenging Disorganization® (ICD®), chronic disorganization (CD) is defined as disorganization that:

- persists over a long period of time
- frequently undermines the daily quality of life
- recurs even with repeated self-help attempts, and
- is expected to continue into the future

In practice, this looks like long-term clutter, painful feelings, and hopelessness. Here are some specific examples of chronically disorganized behaviors and their negative impacts across four key domains: home, work, finances, and personal life.

Chronic Disorganization at Home

Chronic disorganization at home is the most commonly recognized form because its manifestation is most clearly visible. The homes of individuals struggling with CD are typically filled to the max with "things," as are the additional storage spaces they rent when they can no longer fit any more items in their physical dwelling. Because of the physical clutter, these individuals spend inordinate amounts of time looking for lost items, and they have trouble completing basic household chores like cooking or cleaning. The impact on their quality of life is significant because they know they should be completing day-to-day chores, but these tasks are now ten times harder and take significantly more time. This leads to both feeling anxious and neglecting the chores, which creates unsanitary living conditions that ultimately worsen their health. As you can see, it's a domino effect, all leading to a worsened quality of life.

Chronic Disorganization at Work

At work, CD often presents as unreliability and a lack of professionalism. People struggling with CD will perpetually miss deadlines, even small daily ones like showing up for a 10 a.m. meeting. They also frequently misplace important supplies (files or shared supplies in an office, tools and materials in a repair shop, etc.). These organization issues often become so severe that they are ultimately brought to the attention of management, who reprimands, and may even discipline, the worker. Collectively, these actions and their consequences damage the reputation of the individual suffering from CD and may even result in their being fired.

Chronic Disorganization Affecting Finances

Because chronically disorganized people are forever losing bills, invoices, and other essential paperwork, they repeatedly forget to pay bills. This has myriad consequences, including a lower credit score, compounding interest, and accumulating debt. When individuals are trapped in this spiral, they find themselves barely able to afford their current lifestyle, never mind saving money for the future. This can be incredibly detrimental when a house repair is needed, a health scare happens, or even if they just want (but cannot afford) to go on a vacation with friends or family.

Chronic Disorganization Affecting Personal and Social Life

On the outside, people suffering from CD might look like they don't respect themselves or care about others. They will regularly miss outings with family and friends, and they rarely if ever invite anyone into their cluttered homes. They may neglect their own health or hygiene, going for long periods of time without seeing a single health care professional or getting a haircut. This is not because they don't care, but because they have tried and failed to reduce their clutter and improve their lives many times, without success. They see themselves as damaged and beyond help. They've lost all motivation to pursue personal goals, their health is declining, and their personal relationships are fragile or even nonexistent.

This is not a life any of us would want for ourselves. It is not a life any human deserves.

Myths About Chronic Disorganization

Because chronic disorganization is so poorly understood and therefore poorly portrayed in the media, people affected by CD are subject to a lot of incorrect assumptions and stereotypes.

For one thing, people with CD are often assumed to be social hermits who don't want to interact with other humans. This is not true! As you will see in Chapter 3, individuals with CD are often terribly lonely and use belongings to fill the human void in their lives.

Another inaccurate stereotype about people affected by CD is that they're lazy. From the outside, it may look like they don't pick up after themselves or clean their living spaces because they can't be bothered. In fact, it is commonly believed that these individuals aren't troubled by messy spaces or being ungroomed. However, if you lift the hood, you'll find that they hate living in this state of disarray; they are deeply ashamed of it. However, they let it persist because they don't think they deserve anything better, don't know where or how to start, and feel so overwhelmed they become paralyzed.

It is also commonly assumed that if someone's living space isn't obviously, horrifically cluttered, that person isn't affected by CD. This is also untrue. The clutter may be hidden behind closed doors and inside cabinets, and out of sight is not necessarily out of mind. One's state of disorganization is often a matter of perspective. We have worked in homes with little to no visible clutter and in homes so severely cluttered that it's impossible to walk. In both instances, our clients' perception of the clutter is still the same: they hate it, they are ashamed of it, and they find themselves unable to correct it on their own.

Finally, some believe that people with CD are unwilling to change. As a Certified Professional Organizer in Chronic Disorganization®, I want to debunk that myth. People affected by CD do not choose this path. They want help, and it's our responsibility as professional organizers to give them hope.

Diagnosing Chronic Disorganization

So now you know: People who are affected by CD are not people who "love clutter" or simply don't mind living in squalor. In fact, they may have tried many times to get organized and failed. They may be experiencing pressure from friends and family members to "get it together," or they might hear nothing from those important people in their lives because they are hiding away in shame.

Ultimately, there is no one "type" of person affected by CD; it affects people of all ages, races, and classes. However, there are several common contributing factors. These fall into three overarching categories. One category is neurological conditions. People with attention deficit hyperactivity disorder (ADHD), for instance, are susceptible to CD due to an inability to focus and stay on task. Multiple sclerosis patients, on the other hand, are susceptible because of physical limitations due to progressive nerve damage; those whose disease has progressed may be unable to lift or move possessions in order to bring order to their home.

Another category of contributing factors is mental health issues. A severe bout of depression, for instance, can tip an already disorganized person into CD. Unchecked anxiety or obsessive-compulsive disorder (OCD) can do the same.

Finally, a third category of factors is personality traits. Perfectionism, distractibility, and indecisiveness can all contribute to developing CD. These traits alone can't "cause" CD, but they certainly factor in. Tendencies like avoidance and procrastination can also exacerbate things. (For a full list of factors associated with CD, see Appendix A.)

One final note: CD is not something that happens overnight. Many individuals who are chronically disorganized have been so for a long time, possibly since childhood. Therefore, solving the problem will not happen overnight, either. Given the variety of potential causal factors, treating CD often takes time and requires addressing multiple issues. Patience is essential! And most importantly, the treatment you provide needs to be personalized to the individual and the specific challenges they are facing. Identifying these needs and tailoring your approach to fit them is what this book is all about.

What About Hoarding Disorder?

In this book, we're going to treat hoarding disorder as being under the umbrella term of chronic disorganization. It is part and parcel of the same overall problem: a life interrupted and derailed by persistent clutter. In fact, the definition of hoarding disorder presented in the *Diagnostic and Statistical Manual of Mental Disorders* (DSM-5™) has many crossovers with the ICD®'s definition of chronic disorganization; it is simply a more severe manifestation—at the far end of what could be seen as the "chronic disorganization spectrum."

The Clutter–Hoarding Scale®

Such a spectrum has, in fact, been codified by the Institute for Challenging Disorganization® (ICD®). The ICD®'s Clutter–Hoarding Scale® gives professional organizers definitive parameters for evaluating CD. There are five levels that indicate the degree of household clutter or hoarding that a professional organizer might encounter in a home. The levels in the scale are progressive, with Level I indicating a standard household where the organizer does not need any specialized knowledge of CD to be effective, and Level V indicating a household that is extremely unsafe and requires the involvement of a team of professionals to intervene, potentially including mental health professionals, social workers, building managers, and others. (For more information on the ICD® Clutter–Hoarding Scale®, see Appendix B.)

ICD® considers Level III to be the threshold between a cluttered household and one that might be deemed a hoarding environment. Because households labeled Levels III, IV, and V require significant training and experience with individuals experiencing CD, most of the examples I cite in this book will fall into these categories.

Finally, while cases of CD that fall on the farthest end of the spectrum can be easy to identify, not all cases are so clear-cut. If you're ever feeling uncertain about whether a client is suffering from CD, ask the following three questions:

- Has disorganization been a factor in their life for many years?
- Does their level of disorganization interfere with the quality of their daily life or negatively affect their relationships with others?
- Has disorganization persisted despite self-help attempts to get organized?

If the answer to all three questions is yes, they are likely to be experiencing CD. (For a more detailed assessment, visit ChallengingDisorganization.org.)

Finding a Solution

I wrote this book primarily as a professional organizer hoping to help other professional organizers do their jobs more effectively. I saw the shortcomings in the field, leading to the inability of many practitioners to provide lasting change to their clients, and I realized what I was doing with my clients was different. The changes I made stuck. And these changes transformed the lives of my clients for the better.

While I've written this book for my colleagues, I recognize that there will be other readers, such as family members and friends of those affected by CD, who are looking for hope and, ideally, solutions. You are in the right place! While you and your loved one may ultimately need outside expertise, *Making the SHiFT*® will help you better understand what your loved one is experiencing and how you can assist.

Whether you're a professional organizer or simply close to someone struggling with CD, know that this time, your efforts won't be in vain. Together, using the SHiFT® Method, we will break old habits, create new thought patterns, improve behaviors, and bring newfound balance and organization to the lives of people affected by CD.

Chapter 2

Introducing the SHiFT® Method

"Change the way you look at things and the things you look at change."

—*Wayne Dyer*

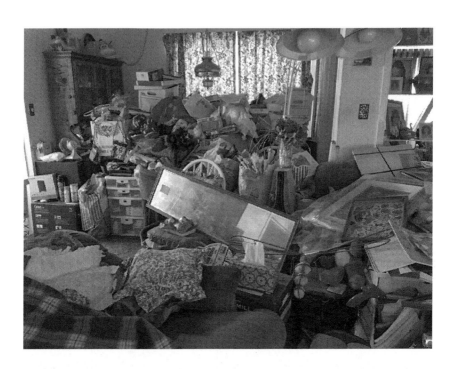

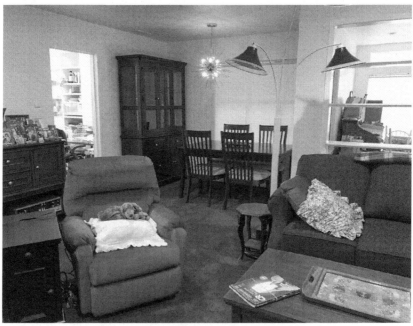

Photo credit: Jen Cazares

Home environments often mirror a person's inner clutter and chaos. Not every element is visually represented, but these two photos show a total transformation in every area of SHiFT®.

Most people with CD have tried, at some point, to get organized. They may even have gotten as far as rearranging or throwing out some of their belongings. Yet these changes rarely stick. Why? Because oftentimes, even with outside help, these individuals are trying to follow conventional organizing methods—and conventional methods don't work for people affected by CD.

Conventional organizing methods rely on logic. Logically oriented people may buy a book about organizing. They may go a step further and hire a professional organizer to help them learn and follow linear organizing strategies. For logically oriented people, these strategies work because their decisions are rational and they can act on well-reasoned logic.

In contrast, people affected by CD might be able to recognize logic, but they don't rely on it to make organization-related decisions; they rely on emotion. Then, because emotion is fickle and rarely matches the logical choice, people with CD often suffer from decision paralysis. As a result, when faced with the question "should I keep this?" they avoid having to decide by keeping everything. This accumulation eventually reaches a point where trying to tackle the clutter creates too much anxiety, and they simply can't do it. Or, rather, they can't do it alone. As coauthors Diane Quintana, CPO-CD, and Jonda Beattie, MEd, share in their book *Filled Up and Overflowing*, "releasing extra stuff for the good of one's mental and emotional health is much easier with an extra set of hands."

You, as a professional organizer, are those extra set of hands. Yet hands alone aren't enough. Even if you help move all the rubbish and excess belongings out of a client's house, it will all come right back if you haven't helped them solve the root of their clutter problem.

That's where the SHiFT® Method comes in.

What Is the SHiFT® Method?

The SHiFT® Method is a nonjudgmental and compassionate approach to helping those who are affected by CD live a fulfilling life without excess clutter. I developed it based on the clear need to address not only a client's physical environment but other essential areas of their life, as well.

The concepts behind the SHiFT® Method were brewing long before I had an acronym to represent them. I knew my CD clients needed more than just decluttering and rearranging their living spaces, and I was doing all sorts of "unconventional" things to help them—I'd just never thought of formalizing what I was doing. What put the seed in my mind was one day, when my friend and fellow organizer Connie Anderson asked to help her brainstorm a TED Talk about people affected by CD. Boy did I have ideas! A few months later, with those ideas still percolating, I attended my high school reunion. There, I saw the acronym PRESENT on a welcome presentation. I loved it! I wanted to come up with something like that to represent my ideas about helping individuals with CD. Fast forward almost six months later: I was organizing paperwork in my office when I picked up my notepad filled with the words and phrases Connie and I had brainstormed. I as I stared at it, the letters started to tilt and merge before my eyes until . . . there! I had it! SHiFT® was born.

Each letter in SHiFT® stands for an aspect of life that is most impacted by CD: **s**ocial connections, physical **h**ealth, mental health ("**i** am deserving"), **f**inances, and **t**ime. In the following chapters you will learn more about what the SHiFT® Method is and how to apply it.

Chapter 3, "S" Is for Social, explores how the SHiFT® Method can help individuals with CD renew and strengthen their social connections.

As social beings, connections make us happy and feel energized. However, when people surround themselves with clutter, they limit their ability to create and nurture relationships with the people they love. The SHiFT® Method helps individuals reduce clutter and make more room, literally and figuratively, for the people they love and care for.

Chapter 4, "H" Is for Health, describes how applying the SHiFT® Method can improve a person's physical health and the health of one's home.

Prioritizing the health of one's home and body is not selfish— it's essential. Moreover, the home and the body are connected. Maintaining a restful sleeping area and sanitary restrooms is paramount to physical health. An organized kitchen is a place for nourishing oneself through healthy eating. Therefore, the SHiFT® Method helps individuals create and maintain a clean home by connecting their living conditions to their physical health in a way that is both motivating and sustainable.

Chapter 5, "i" Is for I am Deserving, examines mental health in connection with the SHiFT® Method.

Chronic disorganization and mental health can often be a chicken-and-egg situation: CD can detrimentally impact one's mental health, while mental health issues can contribute to CD worsening. Self-worth is often the lynchpin, which is why it's the primary focus of the SHiFT® Method. Clients must first believe that they deserve to live a better life before they can take the actions to get them there.

Chapter 6, "F" Is for Finances, provides guidance for taking control over one's finances with the SHiFT® Method.

Without a way to keep track of spending, finances can careen out of control. As debt compounds, stress levels rise. This is a common experience for people with CD because it's hard to keep a handle on finances when paperwork is disorganized, missing, or otherwise hard to find. Furthermore, more spending means more stuff, and more stuff needs somewhere to go, so people with CD often spend even more money on storage units after their homes run out of space. The SHiFT® Method helps individuals learn to take control of their finances, live with less stuff, and reduce their overspending habits in order to reserve their money for doing the things that make them happy.

Chapter 7, "T" Is for Time, helps individuals take back their time using the SHiFT® Method.

Time is a currency no one can earn back. Therefore, time spent moving things around and looking for misplaced items can't be used in more productive, and more enjoyable, ways. The SHiFT® Method helps individuals take back their time and live with intention to create a meaningful, fulfilling life.

The SHiFT® Method is successful because it provides a framework for addressing both the physical and emotional aspects of disorganization in tandem. As a professional organizer, you will learn to address tangible and intangible challenges and organically improve the lives of your clients in a sustainable way. With time, patience, and practice, you will see how applying this method can create a monumental shift in your clients' lives.

How to Use This Book

This book is meant to be practical—something you can use on the job with your chronically disorganized clients. Therefore, while I spend some time explaining concepts and providing background, much of this book is dedicated to exercises you can use directly with the individuals you are assisting and client stories that illustrate how to put the method into practice.

Exercises

In each chapter you will find breakout boxes titled "Thought Box" and "SHiFT® to...."

Thought Boxes pose a question for your client to ponder. You can use these as a discussion aid when you are spending time with clients, or you can even write down the question and have them answer it for homework.

Here's an example:

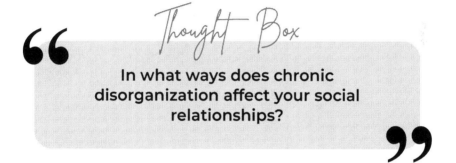

Thought Box

In what ways does chronic disorganization affect your social relationships?

SHiFT® to... breakouts are intended to prompt a new way of thinking. As I tell my clients, "Pretend if you must; just try it on for size." These are important for your client to practice in order to replace old, unhelpful mindsets with outlooks that will help them feel and act deserving of a happy, healthy, uncluttered life.

Here is an example:

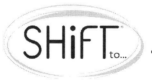

SHiFT to...

telling yourself over and over that you are deserving. Repeat, "I am deserving."

Finally, each SHiFT® chapter ends with a "Think, Write...Deserve" exercise. This is a journal-style exercise that introduces a handful of questions to encourage your client to write down feelings, thoughts, and emotions they may be avoiding. I often introduce these exercises after my client and I have gone through the Thought Box and SHiFT® to... exercises because they build toward this more challenging, introspective exercise.

Here is an example:

Think, Write...Deserve

1. **When and how does loneliness appear in your life?**

2. **What have you tried to overcome loneliness? What has worked? What has not?**

There are five questions in each Think, Write...Deserve exercise.

One more thing: if writing is difficult for your client, you can modify the method to Think, *Talk*...Deserve. If they're comfortable talking through the exercise with you, great; otherwise, encourage them to find a trusted partner with whom they can verbalize their answers.

Client Stories

In addition to providing exercises, I am going to fill the coming chapters with real stories of people whom I have come to know during my years of organizing. (From time to time, my fellow organizer and collaborator Connie Anderson will add a story, too.) Each story is about a client experiencing a positive SHiFT® in the quality of their life.

As you will see, I care deeply about my clients. My role as a professional organizer includes being a trusted confidant, cheerleader, and sounding board. These are not roles I take lightly, and so I use real stories to illustrate their importance as well as to show how to fill such roles effectively. Through these stories, it is my hope that you will learn how applying the SHiFT® Method can lead individuals struggling with CD onto the path toward living full, deserving lives.

Here is the beginning of one client story I will return to throughout the book:

"Patient Zero"

Hank

Meet Hank, one of my first clients suffering from CD who, in a way, helped me form the basis for the SHiFT® Method.

I met Hank after I answered his daughter's plea for help, which came through my website: "*Need cleanup for a very cluttered, hoarded house. Many items have not been moved for many years. Lots of dust, potential mold, three un-house-trained cats. So many house repairs needed it's hard to list them all here, but they have been put off because of the clutter.*"

Although when I met with him, Hank did not self-identify as a hoarder and had never received a formal diagnosis, he met all the criteria in the DSM-5™ for hoarding disorder. His house was in precisely the level of disarray his daughter had described: All the curtains and blinds were closed, and all the lights were turned off. The carpets were saturated with urine and cat feces, which left an overwhelming stench. As I explored the house, the soles of my shoes made crunching or squishing noises with each step. When I finally stopped to put my things down on the floor, Hank quickly said, "I wouldn't do that if I were you."

My initial assessment of the house revealed that not only did Hank have no hot water—the hot water heater had been broken for some time—but both the garbage disposal and the garage door were also broken. Over time, I came to uncover even greater levels of disrepair: the home was overwhelmed with rats, mice, moths, termites, moldy walls, water-damaged ceilings, and so much more.

This house was a high Level IV on the Clutter–Hoarding Scale®, and Hank felt hopeless. He was also elderly and frail. I wondered why he hadn't asked for help before his space devolved into such a horrific condition. As I would learn, it had nothing to do with *who he was* and everything to do with *how he felt*.

Hank's story is not unique. However, as you will see in subsequent chapters, it is a powerful example of how a person's life can improve dramatically using the SHiFT® Method. Hank and others affected by CD can learn to live a deserving, clutter-free life. It just takes a SHiFT®.

Chapter 3

"S" is for Social

SHiFT

"Evolution has placed a bet that the best thing for our brains to do in any spare moment is to get ready to see the world socially... We are built to be social creatures."

—*Vivek H. Murthy, MD,* **Together**

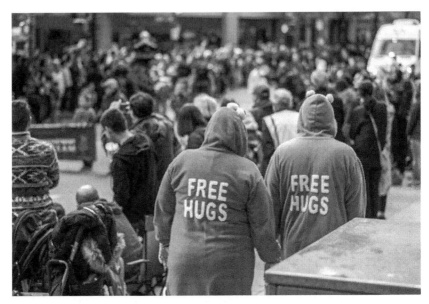

Photo credit: Florian Schmetz, Unsplash

Hugging is one of the most intimate forms of human connection—an essential human need!

Humans have evolved to depend on connection. From the moment we are born, we require not only water, food, and sleep, but also human touch and interaction. As we grow, we develop the desire to belong, to share stories, and to live life with others. Everyone wants to feel included as part of a community, and this is by design. It's how humans have survived for millennia.

Although we quite literally need our family, neighbors, teachers, coworkers, and friends, many of us take our social lives for granted. We assume that whatever anyone's social situation might be, it's what that person wants and has chosen for themselves. Yet for those experiencing CD, this is often not the case at all.

The literal disorganization of someone affected by CD (e.g., a messy house) and the social element of the disorder (the "S" in SHiFT®) can often present a chicken-and-egg problem. Sometimes, a series of fractured social relationships—in some cases precipitated by a neurological condition like ADHD—can lead to feelings of loneliness that the person tries to numb or fill with belongings. In other cases, the excessive, uncontrollable accumulation of belongings can lead to feelings of shame, which causes the individual to shy away from interacting with their friends, family, and community. And of course, both things can be happening simultaneously, as well.

No matter the origin, many individuals experiencing CD are suffering from social isolation. Helping them to SHiFT® their perspective and renew social connections is, therefore, a critical part of setting them on the path to live a full, deserving life.

In this chapter, we will begin by examining loneliness, including the detrimental effects it can have and how those effects compound other issues individuals with CD are experiencing. Then, we will look at ADHD as a contributing factor—how individuals with this condition can easily fall prey to CD and unique approaches that can help them regain their social footing. You will learn to show your clients that one of the best parts of being human is sharing a connection with another human.

> ## *Thought Box*
>
> **Social connections are essential to life. What actions do you take to establish genuine connections with others?**

Loneliness

One might think that between phones, the internet, and social media, loneliness would be a thing of the past. However, research shows that despite these digital connections, humans are getting more and more lonely.

Since the arrival of the COVID-19 pandemic in particular, people are feeling lonelier than ever. According to a 2021 study of over 20,000 adults in more than 100 countries, 21 percent of individuals considered themselves severely lonely, up from 6 percent prior to the pandemic. Results were especially pronounced for those living alone.

Douglas Nemecek, MD, the chief medical officer for the behavioral health division of the pharmaceutical company Cigna, has called the issue of loneliness in America an "epidemic" and has compared its health risks to those of smoking and obesity. This claim can sound hyperbolic, but he may not be far off. According to various studies, a lack of companionship, socializing, and physical contact can lead to mental and physical health issues such as:

- Depression
- Memory loss
- Antisocial behavior
- Cardiovascular disease
- Increase in alcohol or drug use
- Thoughts of suicide
- Dementia

The research is clear: loneliness takes its toll.

How Does Loneliness Affect CD?

No one wants to feel lonely—it's uncomfortable. Some people alleviate this discomfort by consuming alcohol or use drugs.

Some people play video games. Some people get pets. And some people—many of whom ultimately become our clients—deal with loneliness by buying things.

Shopping—or, as many of my clients call it, "collecting"— provides a moment of fulfillment and happiness. But the feeling doesn't last long, and eventually loneliness comes creeping back in, which leads to buying more things. With the endless availability of online shopping, this process is easier than ever. And let's not forget about gifts, heirlooms, and other items that arrive in one's life without any exchange of money at all.

People affected by CD are trying to fill a void in their life, but they are also trying to hold onto personal connection by any means possible. Therefore, letting go of an item that was given to them can feel like letting go of the personal relationship, however strained it may now be. Likewise, letting go of items related to a social activity can feel like giving up a part of their social identity. For instance, let's imagine you have a client who once was an avid fisherman. He loved fishing, he loved the people he fished with, and he loved who he was when he fished. However, when you arrive in his hoarded home, he hasn't fished in years, and the twenty-five fishing rods, fourteen pairs of waders, and boxes upon boxes of line, lures, and hooks are taking up space he doesn't have. These items are imbued with happy memories and even the fantasy of a better future where your client can become that happy fisherman once again. It's painful to let go. Yet these items are merely standing in for the person or the activity that your client truly craves. They're a shadow of the real thing.

> *Thought Box*
>
> **To offset social isolation, how can you connect with friends and family?**

How Does CD Affect Loneliness?

While loneliness can accelerate the onset and severity of CD, CD can also lead to loneliness. The more cluttered a person's home becomes, the more shame they often feel. Shame is a powerful emotion, and people will do many things to avoid it. Shame often leads people affected by CD to shut others out of their home and even their life. It can also cause them to hide in their home, away from others who might judge or look down on them.

I witnessed this shame spiral and how it affected someone starved for social connection with my client, Hank, whom you met in Chapter 2.

Overcoming Shame and Reconnecting with Family

Hank

When we began working together, Hank didn't trust me. All of our early sessions together included his daughter, who had initially reached out to me for help. Later, she shared the fears Hank had harbored when we first began our work: "Who is this stranger in my home? Will she judge me or turn me in to the Adult Protective Services? Is she going to make me throw away my cherished things? Is she going to steal my things?"

Because of those fears, Hank was, quite understandably, quiet and withdrawn during our first several sessions. Yet as our working relationship developed, the emotionless Hank I first met gradually transformed into a different, more engaging person. We eventually started talking, and then we talked some more. Sometimes we didn't even organize his things; we just talked. At first, I was worried that Hank was using lengthy conversations as a diversion tactic to avoid tackling his clutter. However, the more we worked together, the more I understood that listening to what he was telling me during these "chatty" sessions was helping him mentally and emotionally. It also helped me do my job better.

Hank revealed that when he was growing up and even when he attended college, he had had difficulty connecting and fitting in with other people. Even though he joined a fraternity, he did not feel included. He got married in his early twenties and had a daughter, but then his wife cheated on him, and they divorced. He said he wanted to meet another woman and hoped to someday marry again and have more children, but he found that most women didn't seem interested in him. Even his family didn't seem to accept him; two of his sisters lived nearby, yet he virtually never saw them.

Hank's difficulty making and maintaining social connections made him feel increasingly isolated. Eventually, he gave up the search to find a companion. Instead, he adopted cats for companionship and comfort, and he began to accumulate stuff. Living alone in isolation, his home became dark, dingy, and unsanitary. It mirrored how he felt on the inside: worthless and unable to connect with anyone, not even his daughter. Due to Hank's living conditions, his daughter did not feel comfortable or safe enough to bring her daughter—his grandchild—over to visit. He was ashamed that he had let things devolve to this degree, and so he tried to keep even his daughter away. "She's so busy," he would say. What I heard was, "I'm not worth it."

The work to overcome Hank's feelings of worthlessness and renew his social connections was not easy. Months of work turned into years as we transformed his hoarded, dilapidated home into an inviting, livable space. Importantly, we worked not only on clearing his physical space but on helping him recognize and honor his own need for social connection. We conversed, laughed, and, yes, argued at times, and it was incredible to see how those regular social interactions helped the real Hank shine through.

Eventually, Hank was able to entertain his family over a full weekend of socializing and dining, and these visits have now become regular. It took hard work, but Hank found hope by SHiFT®ing his perspective. And as you will see in future chapters, renewing his social connections was just the beginning.

Thought Box

"
How will your life improve once you reduce your household clutter? How will your relationships with your visiting family or friends improve?
"

CD and Loneliness: Which Causes Which?

It's often hard to say which comes first, loneliness or CD. Is it a person's antisocial behavior, poor social skills, and living alone that, over time, leads to CD? Or is it because of the overwhelming clutter and chaotic nature of one's daily living that outsiders are driven away, and loneliness takes hold?

Research once showed that social disconnection was a consequence of hoarding. Now, it is widely believed that social disconnection may be part of the *cause* of hoarding. According to the International Obsessive-Compulsive Disorder (OCD) Foundation, "Loneliness is one of the main factors that causes hoarding to occur." Based on my professional experience, I'm inclined to agree. The perceived need to save, along with the angst associated with discarding things, is simply covering up what's missing in our clients' lives: human connection.

This complex relationship between CD and loneliness is illustrated by the story of another client, Barbara.

Using Hobbies to Renew Human Connection

Barbara

Meet Barbara, a tall, heavyset, eccentric woman with a big heart who chooses not to identify herself as a hoarder but rather as an "obsessive collector with depression."

At least initially, Barbara does not come across as someone who suffers from social isolation. She is a charming woman with a full-time job and myriad interests. However, after one look at her home, it was clear to me that she was affected by CD, which made her lonely.

When we first met, no one was allowed in Barbara's home; she was too embarrassed by the state of her living space to let anyone come visit. Her initial message when she reached out to me was:

Need organizer to help sort and coach me on elimination of excess in storage lockers and home. Hoarder is the most basic term, but I prefer to think of myself as having been an "obsessive collector." Also need resources who can assist to haul away or arrange for pickup of items for donation and can assist with connecting with outlets for items to be financially liquidated, be it consignment, auction, etc. Someone with life coaching expertise would also be helpful, as a part of the decluttering process will involve determining what projects and interests I cannot realistically entertain in the years I have left.

Unlike Hank, Barbara was not living in squalor. Her home, when I first visited, was void of natural light and fresh air, but there were no foul odors. Barbara's excessive quantity of belongings were meticulously labeled. However, seven-foot-high piles of boxes in every room and a lack of walking paths throughout her home qualified it as a hoarded home.

Many of Barbara's belongings related to her hobbies, both current and past. Every time she found a new hobby, she'd dive in headfirst and purchase an astonishing amount of "supplies." For instance, she liked to square dance and therefore owned 100 pairs of boots specifically for square dancing. She also loved to cook and worked part-time at a shop that sold cookware. Every time a new item came to the shop, she was the first one to buy it (with her employee discount, of course). This tendency, I eventually learned, led to her renting a several storage units that she filled with kitchen equipment, some of which she couldn't even use in her household kitchen because the appliance was meant for an industrial kitchen.

In addition to her overabundance of hobby-related items, Barbara also kept more than a few cat towers around her house. It turned out that, like Hank, Barbara had begun substituting animals for human connection and had accumulated more animals than were permitted by the county. Barbara loved her cats, and who could blame her? They were nonjudgmental, loving, and good listeners. Still, pets cannot return a hug, share a laugh, or provide feedback. There is no substitute for human connection.

For Barbara, loneliness played a significant role in intensifying her CD. Therefore, by helping her to overcome loneliness, I was able to also help her make changes that would lessen her hoarding behaviors. Early in our work together, I encouraged her to accept an invitation to volunteer as a pastry judge at a local county fair. Then, I attended the fair to watch her participate. She couldn't believe someone had made the time to come to the event just to see her. I did this so that she would understand that people *do* care about her (I cared about her!) and that her hobbies were not the problem; the problem was her holding on to so many *items* related to the hobbies.

To use her love of cooking to form more human connections, Barbara began helping a friend with her catering business. Meanwhile, to suppress her urge to bring home more feline friends, Barbara started volunteering at a cat rescue center—where, yet again, she could interact with others who shared her interests. In addition, Barbara is now seeing a therapist to talk through her loneliness and depression. I am thankful she chose to pursue therapy, because successfully treating CD is a team effort! The contributions of family, friends, and other professionals are essential to helping individuals overcome loneliness and emerge from their cluttered existence to live full, deserving lives.

Lean into the Human Connection

Hank and Barbara continually bought and kept things to ease their unmet need to feel connected, even if just for a fleeting moment. Therefore, the first step to helping clients affected by CD is to establish a meaningful, supportive connection with them.

Some clients may be aware of the importance of social connections, but many are not. You might be the first outsider to reach out to them in days, months, or even years. It takes time and patience to help those with CD recognize the fundamental need for healthy relationships.

So, how do you do this? You start by taking the initiative to have conversations that create meaningful connection with your clients. When you've become their trusted partner, then you can introduce ways they might reach out and form connections to others in their lives.

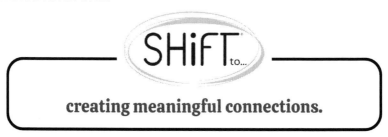

Loneliness is at an all-time high, but that doesn't mean you need to succumb to it. Here are some ways you can connect with people:

- **Call family members or friends you haven't talked to in a while.** In Hank's case, I told him about the benefits of buying a tablet computer. I wanted him to connect with his immediate and extended family by using Facebook. He now stays in touch with his daughter, son-in-law, and granddaughter on a regular basis, and he communicates with extended family members, many of whom he hadn't talked to in over thirty years!

- **Find a pen pal.** Not everyone likes to talk on the phone. If you or your friend or loved one prefer writing, try corresponding via email or even good old postal mail. (Who doesn't love to see a personal letter in their mailbox?) It's a surprisingly intimate way to learn more about others' lives while you share yours.

- **Join online groups that have similar interests to yours.** This is an easy way to connect to and bond with others who share your interests and passions. In Hank's and Barbara's cases, it even led to some in-person engagements with group members who shared Hank's love of gardening and Barbara's love of cooking!

- **Volunteer.** As Barbara discovered, volunteering is a great way to connect with people who share similar interests. Find an organization whose work you are passionate about and commit to a regular schedule of participation.

The Influence of ADHD

Like loneliness, ADHD can also affect CD, and vice versa.

ADHD impacts the way the human brain processes information. Many think ADHD is a children's problem, but in fact, it is a neurological disorder that no one "grows out of." According to the *American Journal of Psychiatry,* 4–5 percent of the adult population in the United States has been diagnosed with ADHD, and this figure is thought to be significantly underreported.

There is no lab test to diagnose ADHD; rather, it involves undergoing professional observation, filling out checklists, and receiving a medical evaluation to rule out other mental or physical problems. This makes ADHD difficult to diagnose, especially because in many cases, the affected individual is the one who must seek out the diagnosis. To do this, they must recognize something is wrong and then follow up with scheduling and attending doctors' appointments—activities that, perhaps ironically, can be difficult for someone with ADHD to do on their own.

How Does ADHD Affect CD?

ADHD can contribute to CD in a variety of ways. ICD® research shows that people with ADHD commonly experience the following:

- Anxiety
- Depression
- Procrastination
- Low motivation
- Forgetfulness
- Poor organizational skills
- Difficulty making deadlines
- Lack of focus or hyperfocusing on tasks
- Problems staying on task and following directions
- Difficulty remembering information and concentrating
- Time management issues

If you recognize certain items on that list as having the potential to worsen social relationships and increase loneliness, you're on the money. Anxiety and depression often diminish social connection because these feelings can cause people to isolate and push others away. Meanwhile, tendencies like forgetfulness or difficulty remembering information and concentrating can make friends and loved ones feel that the person does not care about them, so they ultimately distance themselves.

Items that may not appear to have such a clear connection to worsening social relationships are poor organizational skills, problems staying on task, and time management issues. However, when they contribute to worsening CD—which these do—they absolutely influence social relationships.

Because ADHD brains have trouble concentrating or staying on task, individuals with the condition often leave items out in the open to serve as visual cues. They use this strategy to compensate for an unreliable memory or inadequate time management system, and it does work. When they physically rediscover a bill on the counter, for instance, they are more likely to remember to pay it than if the bill were stored out of sight.

Unfortunately, the more things that are left out, the less chance the person has of noticing—and acting on—them. Eventually, a collection of "visual cues" turns into unmanageable clutter, which then becomes a stressor instead of a solution. The sight of clutter can overwhelm a person with ADHD, and they get trapped in a loop of wanting to organize the clutter but not knowing where to start. This, as you might imagine, contributes heavily to CD.

Think back to Hank. While he was not officially diagnosed as having ADHD or hoarding disorder, Hank possessed many related characteristics that made organizing a challenge. For example, Hank was easily distracted when we were sorting items. Prior to our work together, his distractibility often led to abandoning the task and letting clutter consume his house— which ultimately led to feelings of shame and the devolution of his relationships with friends and family.

Because Hank's short attention span meant he got bored easily, I used various tactics to hold his attention. For instance, I lightened the mood by inventing humorous excuses for saving a particular item. Humor is a great tool to keep a client engaged, and it makes conversations about potentially stressful topics (e.g., getting rid of possessions) feel less fraught. I also used a specific technique to keep his attention focused: I used bedsheets to cover the surrounding area so we could work on one small area of the room at a time without getting sidetracked. I did the same thing when it came to tackling paperwork on his desk—only the relevant items were allowed to remain visible. Of course, this didn't work 100 percent of the time, so I often found myself telling Hank to "stay focused." Don't be afraid to be direct; sometimes that's what is needed!

Directness was certainly called for in the case of Skylar, one of my clients whose undiagnosed ADHD was ruining her business.

CD, ADHD, and Entrepreneurship
Skylar

Meet Skylar, a landscape architect who had owned her own business for over twenty-five years. As many entrepreneurs do, she experienced plenty of ups and downs with her business. However, when I met Skylar, she was on her sixth office manager, her business was on the brink of bankruptcy, and she had already filed for personal bankruptcy three times in the last fifteen years, with a fourth filing on the horizon. It seemed she was having considerably more downs than ups.

Skylar ran her business out of the basement of her rented home. Her office was, in essence, a room with no ventilation, poor lighting, and an absolute mountain of paperwork. When I visited, I quickly realized that her business was struggling because she could not concentrate for long enough to get organized. As we talked through the help I could provide, Skylar could not stay still for a single moment. She perpetually interrupted our conversation to check her computer, take phone calls, and physically wander around the office in a frenzy. I asked if she had been diagnosed with ADHD, and while she said no, her behavior checked all the boxes. I told her this and advised she consult with a mental health professional. After all, it wasn't just her business that was in jeopardy; due to the combination of her ADHD tendencies and her CD, her social relationships were suffering because she spent all her time and energy trying to keep her struggling business afloat.

Unfortunately, not all client stories have a happy ending. Despite my efforts working with her, Skylar could not overcome her hyperactive tendencies. Her business ultimately folded because she failed to get her records in order, invoices paid, and taxes filed. Furthermore, due to lack of ventilation, her residence, including her office, had become infested with mold. A friend told her she needed to get rid of everything in the building, so without consulting me, that's what she did: she rented a dumpster, emptied her entire living and office space into it, and left town.

That was the end of my time working with Skylar. However, years later, I received a message from her. By then she was in her fifties, and she wrote to me, "It never dawned on me that I might have ADHD until you said something. Now I get why I couldn't focus or figure out how to put the pieces of my business together. Thank you for working with me."

It can be difficult for clients to recognize all the factors that are contributing to their CD. Certainly it's not easy to consider that you might have a neurological disorder! However, with patience and diligence, even a story of seeming failure can ultimately be one of success. Skylar might not have been able to revive her business, but she eventually discovered the reason for its failure. I'm hopeful that she has been able to take this knowledge and use it in a way that helps her to live a fuller, more deserving life.

CD, ADHD, and Polyamory

I discovered the intersection of CD, ADHD, and polyamory through my work with two clients, Sue and Cherie. Before I share their stories, I want to provide a disclaimer: what follows is in no way a moralistic judgment of polyamory or anyone who practices it. My assessment here is strictly of my own clients who had both ADHD and CD and who elected to practice polyamory.

As we've discussed, CD and ADHD have a clear connection and, when combined, they contribute to worsening social relationships. In my experience with clients, I've found that CD and ADHD also share connections to polyamory that may not always be in the client's best interest.

Polyamory is the practice of having multiple mutually consensual romantic or sexual partners at the same time. At least one in five Americans has had a consensually non-monogamous relationship at some point in their lives, and about one in twenty is in such a relationship right now. There is little research on the subject, but anecdotally, clinicians share that polyamory is common for people with ADHD.

The intersection between ADHD, CD, and polyamory is this: Individuals with CD alone are unlikely to practice polyamory because they've often cut off all social connection. That's where ADHD comes in. People with CD *and* ADHD have trouble focusing, and so when it comes to romantic relationships, they cannot focus on one partner for long enough for that individual to fulfill all of their needs. Therefore, they engage multiple partners, thus practicing polyamory. Unfortunately, because of their ADHD, the individual has trouble keeping track of and attending to their various partners and relationships. As with their physical belongings, their partnerships become a sort of "collection" that eventually becomes unmanageable.

This lesson about CD, ADHD, and polyamory is one that my client Sue learned for herself.

The CD-ADHD-Polyamory Junction

Sue

Meet Sue, an unmarried woman in her forties who, for as long as she could remember, felt like a "bobblehead": adrift in life with no direction. Never married, unable to commit to a long-term relationship, and incapable of holding a job, Sue was desperate to find answers.

When I met her, Sue was out of a job and had recently come into a small inheritance. She knew she had ADHD, so her first use of the money was to start seeing a therapist. Her second step was to hire me; she wanted to tidy up her small apartment and to organize an off-site storage unit.

In Sue's apartment, mounds of clothes covered the floor, and cat fur coated the clothes, bedding, and furniture. Nevertheless, it seemed like a pretty straightforward job. All I needed were some clothing racks, a dresser, hangers, and some cute baskets. However, as I worked with her to declutter and set up space-saving systems, Sue's seemingly straightforward story became more involved. It turned out that part of her motivation to clean up her space was that she needed to fit her clothes into her new boyfriend's motorhome. She was moving in with him, and they were going to travel across the country. Also, she shared, she was going to try out polyamory.

Before Sue, I had never heard of polyamory. Sue was newly exploring the idea with her boyfriend, who had been living a polyamorous lifestyle for a long time. I had several interesting conversations with Sue, but my learning was cut short when, seemingly out of the blue, she lost her temper, and we ultimately terminated the relationship. The main lesson I learned from this was that it's okay to stop working with a client. As a professional, you need to look out for your own well-being first. The second lesson I learned was to remain compassionate while maintaining healthy boundaries. Sue's anger issues didn't really have anything to do with me; therefore, while I didn't need to subject myself to her abuse, it was acceptable to feel concerned for her and hope she would find the help she needed.

My questions about polyamory remained unanswered until I met a new polyamorous client, Cherie, whom I'll introduce next. However, for Sue, the lifestyle ultimately did not work out. Nine months after we stopped working together, Sue contacted me to share that the road trip had never happened and that she'd broken up with her boyfriend. She apologized for how she'd treated me in our final interaction, and she assured me that she was happier and more grounded now that she'd stopped trying to make polyamory work. I credit Sue's revelation with her getting a handle on her ADHD. If she hadn't, she may have remained untethered, trying and failing to find fulfillment with multiple partners as she wandered across the country. I am hopeful that she remains well and happy today.

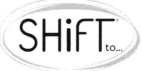

seeing a therapist.

Regular visits to a therapist while working with a professional organizer trained in chronic disorganization can be a very effective method for learning to live a more deserving life.

Connecting ADHD to Polyamory
Cherie

Meet Cherie, a single mother in her fifties who, like Sue, was diagnosed with ADHD and practiced polyamory. Coincidentally, I met Cherie not long after working with

Sue, and my work with Cherie helped to solidify my understanding of polyamory and the role it can play in the lives of those affected by CD and ADHD.

When I met Cherie, she was already practicing polyamory. However, it turned out that the idea had come from her ex-husband. While they were married, Cherie's husband was secretly active in the polyamory community. When Cherie discovered this fact, they divorced. Despite the hurt she felt at her ex-husband's betrayal, however, Cherie became curious about the lifestyle and soon entered into her own polyamorous relationship.

This is the life Cherie was living when she hired me to help her tame the clutter in her house. I could see the influence of her ADHD vividly; it was like a snake eating its tail. Her ADHD caused her to generate clutter (e.g., leaving things out so she'd remember them), which made her more anxious and embarrassed that she couldn't keep her space tidy, and then that stress would intensify her ADHD, which led to more clutter. Our goal was to sort, edit, and organize every room in her house.

As we worked, I was eager to better understand how her ADHD, which was clearly contributing to her CD, impacted her many romantic partnerships. Cherie explained that by living a polyamorous lifestyle, all her needs were being met by different men. No one man could provide her with what she desired emotionally, nor could only one man fulfill her sexually. Yet the more partners she had, the more stress she felt, and the more stress she felt, the less control she had over the clutter in her living space, and the more cluttered her living space became, the less willing she was to have any outsiders come into it, which meant she was spending excess money on hotels and other rentals in order to see all of her partners. She could not seem to stop living in the moment, but living in the moment was wearing her down.

Unfortunately, my story with Cherie also does not have a singular, satisfying ending. We started by organizing her kitchen and got as far as her home office when the COVID-19 pandemic hit. She hasn't yet invited me back, so I don't know whether she continued to practice polyamory, if she got a handle on her ADHD, or how her CD has improved or worsened. I do know that my work with her solidified in my mind the connection between CD, ADHD, and polyamory. It all boils down to the human craving for social connection. Therefore, as professional organizers, we must help our client fulfill this essential human need in a healthy, sustainable way—without resorting to physical *or* relational clutter.

Thought Box

" Visualize having friends over for lunch and having a good time. What feelings would that visit create for you? "

Conclusion

The social lives of the clients we've met so far share a common denominator: The chaos and clutter of their homes are embarrassing for them and keep their family and friends from visiting. As in Hank's case, CD causes their relationships to become estranged, even from those they care about.

In some cases, your client will *appear* to have a flourishing social life: they may be in a romantic relationship (or several), and they may go on outings with others. (This is especially the case for many individuals affected by ADHD—they do not live like hermits!)

Barbara had a job where she worked with colleagues, and she pursued social hobbies like square dancing. Sue and Cherie had plenty of social connections, romantic and otherwise. Yet digging below the surface revealed that their social connections were fractured. Barbara wouldn't let anyone inside her house, Sue struggled with an unstable relationship with her boyfriend, and Cherie was unable to attain lasting satisfaction or fulfillment from any of her multiple relationships. From a social standpoint, these individuals were struggling; you can have social relationships and still feel lonely. And loneliness and CD go hand in hand.

 For these lonely, unfulfilled individuals, social connections are a vital missing component in their lives. Our goal, therefore, is to use the SHiFT® Method to help them manage their CD and strengthen the social component of their lives. We won't necessarily get to see every client through to lasting success. However, every engagement offers an opportunity for learning, and the more we learn, the better equipped we'll be down the line to serve another client who needs our help.

How did Hank, Barbara, and Sue use the "S" in SHiFT® to learn how to live a full, deserving life?

Hank

- Learned how to use Facebook to connect with his family and friends
- Joined similar interest groups on Facebook, taking him out of his comfort zone
- Invited his granddaughter over to bake and decorate cupcakes
- Invited his accountant over for coffee

Barbara

- Accepted an invitation to be a pastry judge at the local county fair
- Started working as an assistant in her friend's catering business
- Volunteered at the cat rescue shelter

Sue

- Began working with a therapist to manage her ADHD and focus on her life goals
- Dissolved a toxic relationship with her boyfriend, realizing she needed to work on her codependent tendencies
- Bought a bus to travel across the country on her own and meet new people along the way

Think, Write...Deserve

1. What's your story of loneliness? Did it begin in your childhood from trauma? Did something discouraging happen at home or at work?

2. How does loneliness show up in your life today?

3. Do you use pets to substitute human connection? How have they changed your feelings of loneliness?

4. If you've found that a cluttered living space damages your relationships with those you love, what have you tried to repair things?

5. Share your moments of victory in overcoming loneliness and restoring relationships that matter to you.

Chapter 4

"H" is for Health

SHiFT

"If you don't make time for your wellness, you will be forced to make time for your illness."

—unknown

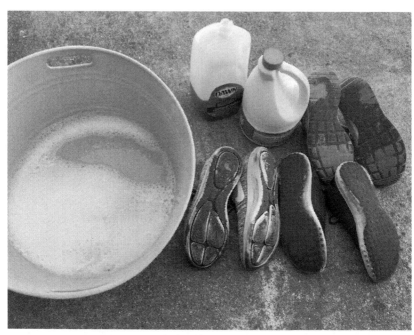

Photo credit: Jen Cazares

***The black gunk on the bottom of my shoes is about
to be scrubbed clean after organizing.***

In 1948, the World Health Organization defined "health" as "a state of complete physical, mental, and social well-being and not merely the absence of disease or infirmity." Put another way, *a healthful lifestyle provides the means to lead a life full of meaning and purpose.*

This definition is still used by health authorities today, and it is highly relevant to our work as organizers. Our purpose is not only to declutter a home, but to create a system the client can use to minimize the clutter that takes away from leading a healthful lifestyle. This is the "H" (health) element of the SHiFT® Method: by helping our clients to improve and sustain their physical health and the health of their home—which are intimately connected—we open the door for them to live full, deserving lives.

Before I dive into physical and then home health, I want to offer a quick disclaimer. I am not a medical professional or a nutritionist. The guidance I offer in this chapter is based on my collaboration with such professionals when helping my clients, my observations when working directly with clients, and my own personal experience. I am aware that environmental changes cannot directly improve all or even most health conditions; yet even the smallest improvements to quality of life are worth it. And as you will see, lifestyle and environmental changes can make a profound difference in some ailments—therefore, it is our responsibility to help our clients try.

Physical Health

Just like loneliness and CD, physical health and CD share a two-way street. On one hand, poor physical health can contribute to CD worsening. If a person is physically unable to take care of themselves or their living space, and especially if they have any tendency to accumulate possessions, it doesn't take long for clutter to happen!

On the other hand, people with CD often neglect their physical health. Sometimes this is intentional—they don't feel worthy, so they neglect themselves, and their health suffers. Sometimes this is the byproduct of living in extreme clutter—they can't cook healthy food because there is no space in their kitchen, they can't exercise because their workout gear is lost in their overfull rooms, and so on. Oftentimes, as you'll see in the case of my next client, Larry, it's both.

On the Move

Larry

Meet Larry, an eighty-year-old divorcée who hired me to help him organize and downsize the house he had lived in for half his life. He was preparing to move to another state where he had more family, and because of his numerous health conditions, he needed help.

By the time I met him, Larry had been diagnosed with a heart condition for which he was prescribed a blood thinner. When he started taking the medication, his doctor took him off of anti-inflammatories and painkillers he had been taking for years for debilitating back pain. A heart attack could kill him, while back pain wouldn't, so from the doctor's perspective, this exchange was logical. However, Larry's quality of life suffered; he spent most days in his La-Z-Boy recliner, trying to find some relief with heating pads.

Meanwhile, Larry ordered virtually everything online. In particular, he owned more clothes than he could ever possibly wear. He would order clothes with the intention of trying them on and sending back whatever didn't fit, but then he would be in too much pain to try them on when they arrived. Eventually, he'd forget what he had bought, discover more clothes to "try," and the cycle would continue.

Larry didn't want to live in a hoarded house. In fact, when he was diagnosed with hoarding disorder years earlier, he went to classes at a local hospital to learn how to curb his hoarding behavior. He learned a lot, but when the classes were over and life events and his deteriorating health got him down, he backslid into old habits. In particular, the death of his thirty-year-old daughter paralyzed him. She owned multiple guitars, thousands of comic books and records, and other entertainment paraphernalia, none of which he could bring himself to touch. In fact, for the twenty years following her death, he maintained payments on two storage units containing exclusively his daughter's belongings without ever visiting either unit. It was only when he decided to move and hired me to help that we were able to finally tackle all of this "stuff."

As we worked together and I discovered the impact Larry's hoarding had on his home environment, I realized the downstream effects of that environment on his deteriorating physical and mental health. The more progress we made in his home and the more praise I heaped on him for maintaining clean, clutter-free spaces, the more Larry's self-esteem improved. Then, the better he felt about himself, the more willing he was to engage in healthful behaviors like cooking fresh food, for example, rather than resorting to takeout.

The most significant indicator that the SHiFT® Method helped Larry make lasting change appeared after we had finished decluttering his house. About six weeks after he sold that house and purchased a new one, he sent me this message:

"My condo is full of boxes and I'm starting to feel like I'm in my old house. I physically can't do much actual unpacking, and my family can't be here every day to help me."

He followed up by asking for my help finding someone local to help him unpack and organize. (Fortunately, my colleague Connie was in his area, and I put them in touch.)

Larry didn't let his physical limitations become an excuse to live in clutter once again; he knew he deserved better! And he knew that to keep his CD at bay, he needed the help of professional organizer. This is the sign of real progress with our clients: when they not only recognize their own need for our help but proactively seek it out.

As Larry's story illustrates, physical health is crucial to maintaining a healthy home. When a client is incapacitated, whether from an illness or accident, the condition of their home can quickly deteriorate. Therefore, this chapter will cover some basics of caring for physical health before moving on to maintaining an environment that promotes health (a healthy home). The three key aspects of physical health I'll address are nutrition, exercise, and medication.

Nutrition

Many individuals affected by CD suffer from poor nutrition. Part of this has to do with the fact that their kitchens are often so cluttered that they have no room to prepare and cook fresh food (we'll get to that a bit later). However, another large influence is a lack of knowledge, along with a degree of gullibility that is shared by much of the general populace.

When I start working with a client and learning about their day-to-day life, I often find that their meals look like one of two things: either they eat prepackaged, ultra-processed, often microwavable food, or they eat takeout. Neither option is nutritious, and the former is particularly lacking. Yet when I talk to my clients, many will insist that they are eating healthfully. "I read the packaging," they'll tell me. "It says it has vitamins! Whole grains!" The mistake they and so many other consumers make is reading the marketing claims on the packaging, rather than the nutrition label. If they looked at the label, and at the ingredients list in particular, they would find myriad unpronounceable words that boil down to three main ingredients: sugar, salt, and fat. No matter what the blurb on the front says, these are not healthy foods!

Now, I'm not villainizing all packaged foods. Precut vegetables (which, technically, are "packaged") can be a lifesaver, and a TV dinner every once in a while is perfectly fine. But when convenience foods make up someone's entire diet, that individual is almost certainly missing out on key nutrients while consuming too much of the salt, sugar, and fat that contribute to diabetes, high blood pressure, and a variety of other health conditions. This is concerning on an individual level, but, as you'll see in the next client story, these poor nutrition patterns don't just affect the individual—they can often extend to an entire family.

Junk Food on Demand

Crystal

Meet Crystal, a married mother of six children ages ten to seventeen. Crystal has a variety of physical and mental health issues that make managing her CD challenging. She has been diagnosed with ADHD, is a recovering alcoholic, and survived a stroke that left her with a slight limp and cognitive issues. She is doing the best she can to manage these maladies, with regular visits to see both a physical therapist and a mental health therapist. However, she ultimately came into my life when her husband and her Alcoholics Anonymous sponsor urged her to get help managing her home and her children.

The home organizing aspect of helping Crystal wound up being pretty straightforward. We created systems for organizing her kitchen, two laundry rooms, master walk-in closet, living room, den, office area, and her children's schoolwork and art supplies. As we organized, I learned her family dynamic: Crystal's husband was the glue holding the household together. He worked full time, managed the essentials of the kids' lives, and golfed on weekends. He also cooked for the family. However, there were no strict mealtimes or rules around food, which ultimately led to a free-for-all.

Because the family was so large and Crystal's husband, the "family cook," was stretched so thin, they kept an industrial-sized refrigerator and freezer in their garage stocked with snacks from Costco. The kids were then at liberty to eat whenever and whatever they wanted. Kids being kids, they grazed on snack foods like chips, boxed mac 'n' cheese, soda, crackers, cookies, and ice cream. In the multiple visits I made to Crystal's house, I never witnessed them consume a single (naturally) green food.

As professional organizers, it's not our place to lecture a client on what they're feeding their children. However, kids learn from their home environment. Crystal's kids were learning poor nutrition habits, *and* they were picking up habits from Crystal's CD. Beyond eating so much processed food, the kids left dirty dishes and snack wrappers all over the house—ultimately contributing to their chaotic, chronically disordered home life.

Unfortunately, I was not hired to go to Crystal's home often enough to give this story a satisfying ending. However, I am choosing to share it as an example of how CD and poor nutrition can go hand in hand, and also as a story you might use to encourage your own clients. Sometimes, even if a client feels undeserving themselves, when they see how their actions are hurting others they love, such as their spouse or children, they will find new resolve.

In addition to consuming too much ultra-processed food, the other eating pattern I frequently see with my CD clients is an abundance of takeout food. Not all takeout food is unhealthy; in fact, today there are more healthy options than ever, now that so many restaurants provide delivery. Yet the problem even with healthier takeout options is the portion sizes. They're enormous! It's not healthy for anyone to eat that much food in one sitting. And yet because it's portrayed as a "single meal," many people consume it all.

The way to solve these two nutrition issues—too much processed food and too much food in general—is to cook whole, unprocessed food. As organizers, we want to raise our clients' awareness of good nutrition practices and to encourage them as they take steps toward cultivating a more healthful diet.

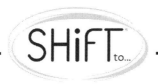

meal planning and prepping.

Planning and prepping meals in advance is one key way to get more home-cooked, nutritious food into your diet.

Not everyone has time (or the desire) to cook a full meal right at lunch- or dinnertime, which is why planning and preparing meals in advance is such a sound strategy. And there are a number of ways to do it! If you enjoy cooking, you can certainly buy all fresh ingredients and prepare them yourself. If that sounds overwhelming, there are myriad shortcuts available. Today, many grocery store items are offered partially prepared: pre-chopped vegetables, pre-peeled fruits, hardboiled eggs, microwavable rice, and the list goes on. There are even meal delivery services like Home Chef and Blue Apron that not only provide recipes and ingredients, they pre-measure the portions of food you're going to cook!

However you do it, the advantage of preparing food in advance is that when it's available in the refrigerator, ready to be assembled or heated up, it becomes just as convenient as takeout or frozen dinners, and now you're nourishing your body. Furthermore, planning and prepping your meals saves you time—by eliminating the need to decide what to make and trips back and forth to the grocery store—and money—because takeout is expensive!

Follow these easy steps:

1. Choose a few recipes you'd like to try for a week of healthy meals.

2. Make a complete list of ingredients.

3. Shop on one day for everything you need.

4. Prep your meals for the week.

Exercise

Good nutrition is essential to good physical health, but on its own, it can only do so much. Another key element is exercise.

Many people—CD clients included—are resistant to exercise. "I don't have time" or "I don't have the right equipment" or even "I don't like to sweat" are excuses we've all heard and maybe even offered up ourselves. That's why, when I work with clients, I try to refer to exercise as "physical activity" or even just "being active." I want this aspect of health to be approachable and achievable because it's very important.

Being active has numerous health benefits, both physical and mental. It can improve sleep quality, energy levels, mood, and memory, while reducing feelings of anxiety and depression. It can even help you live longer! The bottom line is that exercise improves nearly every aspect of health.

The process of performing dedicated physical activity every day can also help to manage CD. Committing to any type of regular physical activity helps clients build a routine into their day, which in turn helps them to feel a sense of control. For someone who often feels helpless and uncertain, even the slightest feeling of control can be game-changing. They start to learn to feel deserving (the "i" in SHiFT®) because they are learning that they can depend on themselves. And in the meantime, they're doing something that makes their body and brain healthier (the "H" in SHiFT®). It's a win-win.

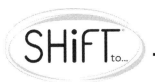

adding more activity into your daily routine.

Increasing your daily activity doesn't have to mean buying an expensive gym membership, preparing to run a marathon, or even owning home exercise equipment. Pick a way you like to move your body—something you really enjoy. Make it as simple as you like; it should be something you can do at home at no or little cost, even without equipment, if that's your preference. Walking, dancing to your favorite music, marching in place, whatever it is that will get your blood flowing and fresh air circulating for at least 20 minutes a day, will do the job. Plus, as an added bonus, forms of exercising like taking a walk around the neighborhood or finding a favorite local park can be done with a friend or in a group—a great way to build and sustain healthy social relationships (the "S" in SHiFT).

In addition to scheduling regular physical activity, there are also tiny daily changes you can make to be more active. Instead of taking the elevator, take the stairs. Instead of searching for the closest parking spot at the grocery store, find one farther away. No matter what the activity is, every bit of movement adds up and will make a difference to your overall health.

Medication

One thing that has surprised me as I visit more and more cluttered homes is the abundance of drugs I encounter. By "drugs," I mean everything from ibuprofen to antibiotics to marijuana. Clients with CD often have intersecting health issues and can be on as many as five or more drugs, prescribed or otherwise.

There's not much we can do regarding clients' recreational drug use other than to educate them on the potential risks. However, when it comes to prescription medication, a crucial task where clients need our help is organizing the medications they are supposed to take. I often create a list of medications, including the doctor who prescribed that medication and that doctor's phone number, so that my client can easily keep track of what they are taking and when they're supposed to take it, and they can call for a refill when something is running out. Some clients will even grant me permission to collaborate with their medical and mental health providers. This approach is ideal because it allows me to dive deeper into supporting them. I'm often able to help these professionals, who never see the inside of the client's living space, to understand some of the challenges that client is facing and to recognize if they are (or are not) making progress.

Of course, while taking medications on their prescribed schedule can help improve a client's health, no medication can make up for poor nutrition or lack of exercise. That's why the best possible result comes from a combination of all three physical health approaches. As your client begins to eat more nutritious food, move their body more often, and regularly take their medications, you may find that, over time, their doctors will wean them off of some medications. This is a clear-cut sign that their physical health is improving—they no longer need a medication to prop up a crucial bodily function! Therefore, always approach a client's physical health using this three-pronged approach: nutrition, exercise, and medication.

Missing Medications
Don

Meet Don, a divorced father of two adult children who lived in a three-bedroom, split-level condo.

Don originally hired me to help him get files in order. He'd inherited several businesses from his father, who had had a stroke, and he was trying (and failing) to convert the bookkeeping from analog to digital. However, it quickly became apparent that Don needed assistance that went beyond paperwork.

Don told me that when he was a child, he had been diagnosed with ADHD. He suffered from depression, obesity, drug addiction, traumatic brain injury (TBI), and narcolepsy. His relationship with his father both before and after the stroke was volatile, and he had been a victim of domestic violence during his married years.

All of these factors added up to Don feeling unworthy (which we'll return to in the next chapter) and increasingly neglecting his personal health and the health of his home. Although he told me that he was trying to stay on top of the daily business operations and maintain his health, he recognized he was not succeeding.

As we began organizing, I broached the topics of nutrition and exercise. Don pointed out that he had just purchased a Peloton (stationary) bike. However, when I finally located it in his bedroom, I discovered it had been repurposed as a clothes hanger. Don knew he needed to exercise; as we unearthed the bike, he told me, "I wear a 3X, I don't want to wear a 4X!" On a subsequent visit, I discovered that the Peloton bike had been moved out of his bedroom, into a second bedroom he called the "storage room." That room was packed with stuff and barely had space for the bike. While he had made the effort to move the bike, Don was still not using it to exercise.

As I worked on decluttering and sorting the rest of Don's house, I learned that medication was a challenge for Don on two fronts. First, he had prescription medications that he was not successfully managing. During our early days of organizing, he would send me text messages that he was "tearing the house apart trying to find medicine for his TBI." This regular "tearing apart" of the house did not make it easy to tidy, and it certainly did not help him keep areas we had organized tidy. Second, Don had a huge quantity of over-the-counter medicines and first aid supplies that were strewn all over the house. When

I asked him about this, he said he could never find what he needed, so he just ordered more.

Where we failed initially with the Peloton bike, we succeeded with the medications. Using the app Airtable, I inventoried all of Don's medicines and first aid supplies so he'd know exactly what he had on hand. I turned his linen closet into a "pharmacy"—a one-stop shop for all his medicines and first aid supplies. Then, I created small, manageable first aid kits for each room of the house. When the kits ran out of items, Don would refill them from his "pharmacy closet."

This plan may not work for everyone, but it worked well for Don. He thought the whole system was brilliant and was pleased by an added silver lining: since he no longer feared running out of medication, we could turn off many of his auto-renew orders from Amazon. Now he was saving money, too!

Home Health

Eating nutritious food, exercising regularly, and taking prescribed medications correctly are essential actions for keeping the body healthy. But physical and mental health are affected by more than just behaviors—they're affected by environment. That is why, in this chapter about health, we must address home health: the cleanliness, utility, and invitingness of one's home.

Thought Box

If you were to describe a healthy home for you and your family, what would it look like?

One surefire way to assess a client's home health is through the lens of cleanliness. Imagine living in a home infested with black mold spores, rat droppings, rodent carcasses, half-inch-thick layers of dust, and a forty-year-old carpet saturated with pet urine. This doesn't sound like a very healthy home, does it? It certainly doesn't sound like a place where someone's body and brain would be able to stay healthy. Yet this is exactly the home in which Hank, whom you'll remember from the last few chapters, was living.

Repairing Home Health to Restore Physical Health

Hank

Hank's home was literally making him sick. Between the mold, rat excrement, dust, and pet urine, it should be no surprise that Hank had developed chronic respiratory problems by the time I met him. He'd gone to see his doctor many times, but she had no idea of the toxic air Hank was inhaling every day. Therefore, the doctor would prescribe an inhaler and antibiotics, which helped in the short term, but soon Hank would be back in her office with the same symptoms. It was a vicious cycle.

To make matters worse, Hank's hygiene was abysmal. His hot water heater had been broken for years, so he had resorted to heating water on the stove for sponge baths. Without hot water, he was also unable to clean his dirty dishes, which he instead stacked all over his kitchen, prohibiting cooking and attracting insects and rodents.

Eventually, I got a hot water heater installed for him and cleared the kitchen of dirty dishes. (Dish washing alone took me and a partner *four hours*.) Next, I hired a hauler and began to purge the house of items that had been compromised by water damage, dust, pet urine, termite infestations, and mold. My organizing partner and I carted away fifteen truckloads of expired food, damaged books, broken furniture, old newspapers, and moldy linens. When we finally cleared the hoarded piles, we made a discovery: the condition of the floors, walls, and the structure of the home made it unsafe to live in. The house needed to be repaired and remodeled.

For Hank, who had lived in the same home for fifty years—and had barely stepped outside in the last thirty—this repair and remodel job presented a potentially traumatic disruption. I discussed it with him at length, weighing all of the pros and cons. Eventually, buoyed by the possibility that his family would one day stay in his home with him (while currently, they refused to even visit), Hank agreed to move forward.

Initially I tried to keep Hank in his home. I instructed the contractor to begin work in two rooms that could be closed off from the rest of the house, so Hank and his two cats could remain living in the rest of the home undisturbed. However, after those two rooms were completed, I realized that the only way the house could finish being remodeled was if Hank moved out.

Moving out of his home of fifty years, even temporarily, was emotionally difficult for Hank. In fact, this type of move is so emotionally difficult for anyone affected by hoarding disorder that when I asked two of the country's top hoarding experts, Dorothy Breininger and Matt Paxton—perhaps best known for their work on the A&E television show *Hoarders*—neither had ever heard of a hoarding client who voluntarily moved out to have their home remodeled.

But Hank did it. For six months, Hank and his cats lived in a small temporary home nearby while his home was remodeled. When he would start to get anxious, I applauded his bravery and reminded him that this arrangement would not last forever. I explained that when he moved back into his home, it would be a healthy home where his granddaughter, daughter, and son-in-law could visit and maybe even spend the night.

While construction was in progress, I took him shopping to find replacement furniture: a bed and dresser for his bedroom, plus a hide-a-bed for his daughter and son-in-law and a bed for his granddaughter. We bought a new dining room table, upon which I encouraged him to imagine serving a meal to his family. We purchased a couch, recliner, and living room chairs where I told him his family could soon be sitting. Giving him this happy vision of the future helped Hank soldier on, even when he was desperate to be back in his home. He was worthy of having a healthy home where his family could visit, and he was beginning to believe it.

Another way to assess home health is to look at it in terms of safety. Through a professional organizer lens, the technique for improving the safety of a home is called Harm Reduction Theory. According to the Institute for Challenging Disorganization® (ICD®), Harm Reduction Theory improves a client's general health by decreasing the compulsive hoarding elements in their living environment. This includes critical changes like clearing walkways in the home to accommodate an ambulance gurney, as well as other, less dramatic examples like assuring exterior doorways and windows are accessible, removing tripping hazards to reduce the risk of falls, and addressing fire hazards.

When you're assessing what needs to be done to perform harm reduction in a home, a good place to start is with the client's physical abilities or limitations. If they're at risk of falls, for example, then belongings strewn around the floor are a hazard. Other safety considerations are universal. A ceiling-high tower of precariously stacked boxes will threaten anyone's safety!

Creating a Safer Home
Barbara

When I first began working with Barbara, whom you'll remember from Chapter 3, she was about to undergo surgery. Therefore, I spent the six weeks before her surgery making sure she would have a safer home to return to post surgery.

One area of focus was mobility. If you recall, Barbara's home was absolutely packed with "stuff" to the point where she couldn't use her kitchen, couldn't sit in her living room, and could barely walk anywhere. In the weeks leading up to her surgery, I cleared pathways between the rooms of her house and then gathered discarded items to donate. The goal was to ensure Barbara had more space to safely maneuver around her home when she returned from surgery.

The other primary safety risk I addressed was the risk of falling objects, specifically in her living room. Barbara's living room had vaulted ceilings, which enabled her to stack boxes as high as she could reach. On average, these stacks were eight boxes high and posed a serious threat of toppling over and hurting Barbara. What's more, I noticed that her cats liked to playfully jump among the towers of boxes. When I asked Barbara if she had ever heard the term "flat cat," she said no. I explained that when cats play among heavy piles of boxes, they could knock a pile over, which might fall and crush them. This helped to persuade Barbara that we needed to address her towering living room piles. She cared about her own health, of course, but she absolutely couldn't bear the thought of a beloved cat being harmed!

> **Do you believe that a healthful house matters to your physical and mental well-being? Can you explain why?**

The final way of assessing home health is to determine whether a client is able to use the rooms in their home for their intended purpose. The square footage is irrelevant; whether the home is a studio apartment or a mansion, the zones in a home are intended to support specific essential daily living activities. Kitchens are for cooking and eating. Bedrooms are for sleeping. Bathrooms are for personal hygiene. If your client is struggling to use any of these rooms for their intended purposes, it will affect their physical and mental health in negative ways.

Kitchen

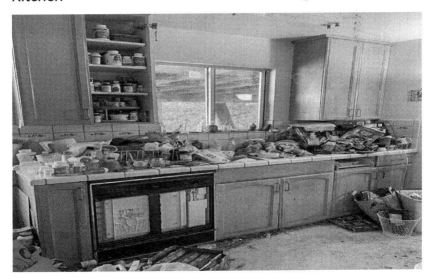

Photo credit: Jen Cazares

Having this much clutter makes it very challenging to prepare a healthy meal.

I see the kitchen as the heart of the home. It's a communal space where family and loved ones can come together, and it's also where meals are prepared to fuel and nourish the home's occupants, as well as loved ones they have invited inside.

For this reason, I've found that the condition of the kitchen says a lot about the health of the client. When I open a pantry door, I typically see it filled with overly processed prepackaged foods. When I open a refrigerator and freezer, they, too, are often filled with unhealthy convenience foods. This is not a coincidence; these foods are cheap to buy and easy to prepare. You don't need a stove or even a plate—all you need is a microwave, and voilà! Dinner is served!

A large reason convenience and simplicity are the most prevalent features of our CD clients' diets is that many clients' countertops—and kitchen tables, and stovetops—are too cluttered to use. It's easy to settle for unhealthy food when there is literally no surface upon which to set a bowl, pot, or cutting board. And while certain appliances may have been purchased with healthier eating in mind, they need to be accessible to contribute to a healthier diet. You can't toast bread if you can't find your toaster. You can't make a smoothie if your blender is buried. You can't even plug in an electric kettle if the outlet is obscured by a mountain of other belongings.

Thought Box

66

What does an organized kitchen look like to you, and how would this kitchen serve you better?

99

Clearly the state of the kitchen affects the quality of food a person can prepare, and the quality of the food affects that person's health. But the state of the kitchen also affects other behaviors that contribute to healthy eating and social well-being.

For instance, making a seat at the kitchen table for every member of the family (even a family of one!) is important. From a health standpoint, sitting at the table to eat helps to prevent overeating. The more mindless a person is when they eat, the more they tend to eat—and what is more mindless than eating on the couch in front of the television? Therefore, the place to eat regular meals is at the kitchen table, not the couch.

Of course, kitchen tables are often used for a variety of purposes—and that's OK. During the day, the table can serve as a temporary multifunctional workspace; however, when it's time to eat, I coach my clients to clear the table and honor its primary purpose: a place where family and friends gather for social interaction and physical nourishment.

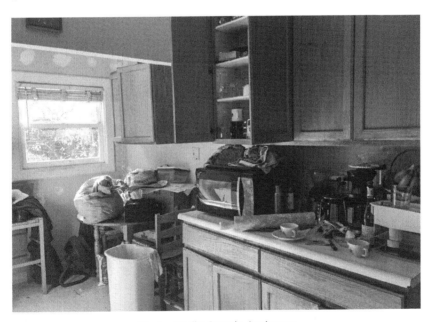

Photo credit: Connie Anderson

This family hadn't eaten together for over a year due to the stagnant clutter on the kitchen table.

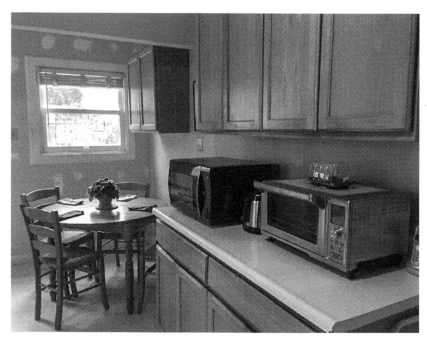

Photo credit: Connie Anderson

By setting a goal for a healthier lifestyle, this family cleared their kitchen clutter and were finally able to eat together once again.

Bedroom

Good sleep is essential to health, which is why we have bedrooms: they're meant to facilitate a regular, restful night's sleep. Unfortunately, CD often thwarts this essential function.

Some clients cannot even reach their bedroom because the staircases and hallways leading to it are blocked by belongings. Other clients who are able make it to their bedroom don't bother because their bed is unreachable (the bedroom is too full of stuff) or unavailable (the bed is piled with so much stuff that they can't sleep in it). And finally, even if there is a space large enough on the bed to lie down, many clients don't want to because their mattress is decades old, the sheets are filthy, and everything is infested with bed mites and even fleas. It's not a healthy room!

Here is a brief example of how liberating it can feel for someone affected by CD to be able to simply lie down in their own clean, cleared bed.

The Cycle of Thrifting

Colt

Meet Colt, an elderly single man recovering from a stroke. Because of the stroke, Colt has limited use of his right arm and difficulty with balance. When things fall on the floor, they tend to stay there. The stroke also makes climbing the stairs to his bedroom difficult, so when Connie and I met him, Colt was sleeping in his recliner downstairs instead.

Colt hired us for several reasons. For one thing, his love of thrifting—which includes capitalizing on coupons and senior discounts—had become a problem. He loved collecting coins, DVDs, and quirky bric-a-brac like tribal shrunken heads; however, the more stuff he brought home, the less space there was to move around his condo. Tripping hazards were around every corner, and he needed help.

Colt also hired us because he needed income. His stroke had left him unable to work, and the disability support he received wasn't enough. Fortunately, he had amassed a substantial quantity of collectible coins that filled scores of boxes scattered around the house. He needed help gathering, sorting, and selling these coins. That's where we would come in.

Finally, Colt hired Connie and me for a very immediate reason: he needed to prepare his condo for a site visit from his social worker. He was concerned, and rightly so, that the social worker would deem him unable to care for himself and force him to move to an assisted living home, which he absolutely did not want to do.

In short, our work with Colt was a success. We organized his home, sold many coins, and helped him pass the social worker visit. But the achievement I want to highlight is the day we were able to clear the clutter—along with an immeasurable amount of cat hair—from Colt's bed. We changed his sheets; it was the first time since his stroke that he had had clean bedding. We drew the curtains back to let in natural light and give him the opportunity to open the windows. The room seemed to breathe new life. It was a healthy bedroom, and Colt loved it. By reclaiming his home, and especially his bedroom, Colt felt a sense of renewed hope and optimism. He was learning to feel deserving.

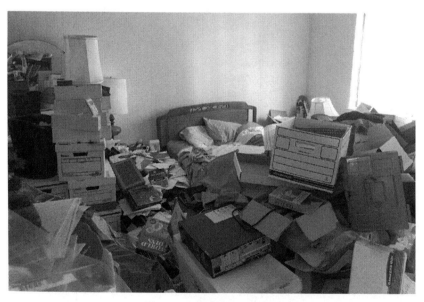

Photo credit: Jen Cazares

Can you find the bed in this photo? Instead of sleeping in his bed, Colt slept in his recliner.

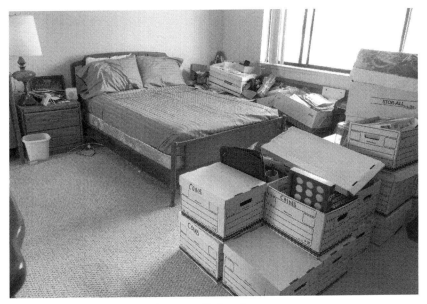

Photo credit: Jen Cazares

Colt's bedroom—now a healthy room that's light and airy—and his bed with fresh, clean sheets.

Thought Box

> " What can you do to better maintain your home environment? How can you keep it in working order and free of clutter, dust, pet hair, spider webs, etc.? "

Bathroom

We have, at last, arrived at the room most essential for hygiene: the bathroom. Bathrooms are meant for bathing, brushing teeth, and using the toilet. Yet none of these tasks can be accomplished—at least easily or effectively—if the bathroom is unreachable or unusable.

When you visit a client's home, check: Does the toilet flush? Does warm water flow from the shower and sink? Are the counters, cabinets, and basins free of dust? A "no" to any (or certainly all) of these questions may indicate a lack of use. And if your client isn't regularly using their bathroom for its intended purpose, you can be fairly certain their health is suffering as a consequence.

Developing Accountability
Fiona

As shared by Connie Anderson

Meet Fiona, a diagnosed paranoid schizophrenic in her early fifties who was very much on her own. Her only remaining family was her ninety-two-year-old mother who lived in a nursing home. She had a part-time job as a mail sorter for a large corporation, but outside of work and visiting her mother, Fiona's social interactions were limited.

Fiona became my client when her fiduciary reached out. When I arrived at her home, one of the first health hurdles I was determined to help her overcome was the hurdle of using her bathroom.

Fiona was among several clients who were not only actively avoiding using their bathroom but had done so for years. This is not to say she had no hygiene practices at all; people who avoid their bathrooms will typically find alternative places to perform the necessary activities. For instance, Fiona was using her kitchen sink to brush her teeth, and she used a washcloth to give herself a sponge bath since her bathtub was filled with items.

To help Fiona transition back to using her bathroom for its intended purpose, I helped her organize it and hired a cleaner to come in and get rid of the grime.

Then I created a chore chart to help her stay on a regular maintenance schedule. She ultimately shared the chart with her therapist, which helped immensely because, now that she had to check in with her therapist about the chart, she gained accountability. I highly recommend this approach for clients who are working with mental health and/or social work professionals. The more they share the organizing methods you've helped them develop with other members of their support system, the more accountable they become!

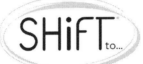

SHiFT to...

asking for help to achieve what you want to accomplish.

Finally, a bathroom that *is* being used but is not clean or organized is of equal concern. Bathroom countertops, medicine cabinets, cabinets under the sink, and closets can quickly become so cluttered that the individual affected by CD can never find what they need. This often leads to accumulating duplicate items, which add to the clutter.

Additionally, bathrooms, like kitchens, are highly susceptible to bacteria, mold, and grime. This is even more of an issue for clients who own cats. Bathrooms are the obvious place to store litter boxes, and more cats means more litter boxes that not only need to be cleaned but that release dust and grit onto surrounding surfaces.

Cleaning and organizing their bathroom will help your client maintain good hygiene—and therefore better health—but remember: making this setup sustainable is essential. For Fiona, creating a chore chart helped, and sharing that chart with her therapist helped even more. For others, hiring a professional cleaning service or housekeeper may be the solution. Work with your client to determine what will work best for them. This can take time, but it's time well spent!

Conclusion

Health is essential to living a full, deserving life. Yet health is affected by many "inputs," from the food one eats to the state of one's bedroom. As we saw in the client stories in this chapter, physical health is interconnected with home health in a symbiotic way. A person needs physical health to care for their home, but, as in Hank's case, a cluttered, unsanitary, dust- and disease-ridden home can worsen physical health, which in turn worsens the health of the home.

This is why it is our responsibility to use the SHiFT® Method to look at the full picture of our clients' health. Are they eating nutritious food? Exercising regularly? Keeping track of their medications? Are they able to cook in their kitchen, sleep in their bed, and care for their hygiene in a clean, functional bathroom? By evaluating these areas of health, we can help our clients become well, both physically and mentally, and maintain a home that supports their health.

How did Larry, Crystal, Don, Hank, Colt, and Fiona use the "H" in SHiFT® to learn how to live a full, deserving life?

Larry

- Began cooking real food in his clutter-free kitchen
- Asked for help getting organized after he moved to prevent backsliding into hoarding behaviors

Crystal

- Works out on a regular basis
- Hired a housekeeper to come three times a week
- Regularly sees her therapist
- Works on being a good role model for her children

Don

- Tried a weekly food delivery service in order to eat fresh vegetables
- Made space in his bedroom to re-introduce exercising on the Peloton bike
- Designated an accountability partner (in this case, me) to keep his commitments

Hank

- Allowed his compromised furniture to be hauled away
- Hired a housekeeper to clean regularly

Colt

- Transitioned to sleeping in his clutter-free bed
- Curbed his thrift store shopping and donated excess items

Fiona

- Hired a house cleaner to deep-clean the kitchen and bathroom
- Enlisted her therapist to help her stay accountable for completing her weekly home maintenance tasks
- Began brushing her teeth and showering daily in her bathroom

Think, Write...Deserve

1. What are you doing to live a healthy lifestyle (e.g., gym workouts, walks with friends, planning your meal schedule, hiring a housekeeper)?

2. Accountability is important for staying focused on living a healthy lifestyle. How are you staying accountable?

3. Do you believe it's important to live in a healthy home? What does a healthy home look like to you?

4. What was your home like where you grew up? How about your meals? Describe your childhood home and meals, and follow up with what you may or may not like to do differently now that you have autonomy over these aspects of your life.

5. With respect to improving your current health and your environment, what should you *stop* doing?

Chapter 5

"i" is for I Am Deserving

SH**i**FT

"Sometimes the hardest part of the journey is believing you're worthy of the trip."

—Glenn Beck

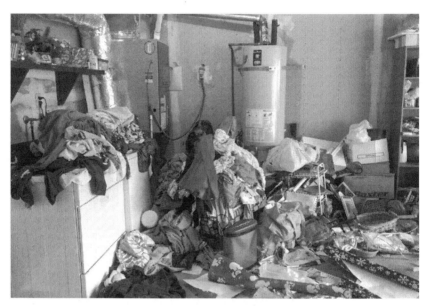

Photo credit: Jen Cazares

Backlogged laundry and other items spread all over the garage.

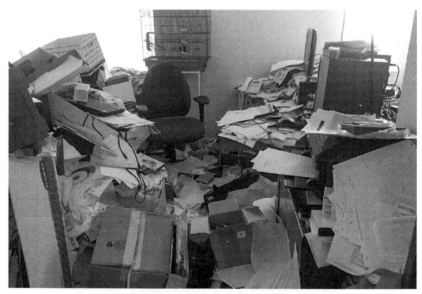

Photo credit: Connie Anderson

A home office in need of attention.

When I introduce the SHiFT® Method, one of the first questions I'm often asked is, "Is the 'i' supposed to be lowercase?" The short answer is yes, this decision was intentional. Once I explain it, you'll see why.

Stop and really look at the word:

SHiFT

Now pretend it's a piece of art—a collection of shapes, rather than a collection of letters. Which shape draws your attention? I suspect it's the one in the middle. What does that shape remind you of?

To me, the lowercase "i" looks like a little person. It represents the human at the center of the SHiFT® Method, the client. They're surrounded by all these other life factors—social factors, health, finances, and time. When these other factors start to seem overwhelming, the human ("i") at the center gets crushed.

SHiFT

By helping your client to reframe their outlook and learn to manage the social, health, financial, and time management aspects of their life, the S, H, F, and T back off. More space is created, and your client finally has room to breathe, experience happiness, and even feel deserving of that happiness.

SHiFT

The "i" in the SHiFT® acronym stands for "I am deserving." To make lasting, positive changes in their life, a person affected by CD must feel deserving of those changes. It's why organizing for the sake of organizing doesn't work with our clients—if they don't feel like they deserve to live in a nicer home and eat good food and enjoy the company of friends and family, clutter will creep back in and prove their underlying belief: *See? I knew I didn't deserve a better life*.

But they *do* deserve a better life. Everyone does. So this chapter, which I consider the heart of the SHiFT® Method, is about gently helping our clients recognize—and embrace—this simple truth.

"Stuff" and Self-Worth

It can be logical to wonder: If someone thinks they don't deserve anything nice, why do they buy so much stuff? This is a conversation I sometimes have with those outside of professional organizing, when I am explaining what's at the root of why my clients need help. Cultural ideas like "I earned this" and "I deserve a treat" are so prevalent that we think if someone feels undeserving, surely they wouldn't treat themselves. So, for the moment, let's replace the word "deservingness" with "self-esteem."

We've all known someone with low self-esteem. Think of someone you know (or knew) and then remember the ways they overcompensated. Maybe you're recalling the girl in high school who felt insecure and wore tons of jewelry and makeup in an attempt to cover up that insecurity. Maybe you remember the boy in college who felt like a misfit, so he binge-drank and smoked even though he didn't really enjoy either activity. Maybe you're thinking of the colleague who is so unsure of their own skill level that they make entirely unrealistic claims on social media.

Some people affected by CD act similarly. Their low self-esteem makes them feel like they aren't worthy of anyone's time, attention, or affection for simply being who they are, so they buy a whole bunch of stuff to impress others and feel more accepted and liked. If you remember Barbara's story in Chapter 3, that's something she did. Barbara wanted to be accepted and admired by fellow cooking hobbyists, so she was always the first to buy a new appliance, dish, or ingredient as soon as it was available, whether she needed (or ever used) the item or not.

Barbara was a lovely woman. Others would have liked her just fine without her jam-packed kitchen or storage units full of cookware. But she didn't feel that inside. She didn't feel deserving, so she just kept accumulating stuff, trying in vain to fill that hole in her self-worth.

Now, poor self-worth isn't the motivation behind *every* client's CD. As with any mental health condition, no two CD clients are ever the same! For instance, I've seen some clients hoard craft supplies because it's their way of preserving their identity as a creative, crafty person. Never mind that they've only ever made one bracelet or have never completed a painting; as long as they have all of the beads, strings, paints, and brushes (and plenty of them), they feel satisfied that they are a jewelry maker and a painter. Those belongings protect their sense of identity.

For yet other clients, CD itself erodes their self-worth. Just like the "chicken or egg" problem inherent in the Social and Health elements of SHiFT®, "I am deserving" follows the same pattern. In many cases, as their living conditions deteriorate, the person affected by CD feels more isolated and less deserving of a full, happy life. Thoughts like "I can't even keep my house in order" or "No wonder no one likes me, this place is such a mess" creep in, and the person becomes locked in a vicious cycle: they don't feel deserving because their home is such a wreck, but they can't clean up their home because they don't feel like they deserve a nicer living space. They need someone to break the cycle. That's where we come in.

Cleanouts Don't Work; Compassion Does

Feeling worthy and deserving is essential to decluttering because it's what makes this new way of living "stick." This is why our work as professional organizers goes beyond superficial organizing: because if it were just about "getting organized," cleanouts would work. And experts agree that they don't.

A cleanout is, essentially, an intense purge and reorganization of a space, room, or entire home, often performed by an outsider (i.e., not the person living in the home). Speed and efficiency are priorities in a cleanout, with the rationale often being "let's rip this Band-Aid off."

Yet according to the International Obsessive-Compulsive Disorder Foundation (IOCDF), cleaning out a hoarded home without the involvement of the person affected by the disorder rarely works. The reason is that when the organizer leaves, they're leaving the same person with the same problems and feelings alone in that spick-and-span house. The client had no say in what stayed and what went, so they're inclined to replace the discarded items to refill the void and rebuild the wall of emotional protection those items provided. In no time at all, things are back to the way they were, and everyone—included the person who was supposed to have been "helped" by the cleanout—is feeling frustrated and often defeated.

Why Cleanouts Fail

Cleanouts fail on three counts. First, the organizer neglects to give the person affected with CD the *tools* to manage their new, clean space. (Think about it: if the client had the knowledge and skills to stay organized, they wouldn't have needed a cleanout in the first place!)

Second, the organizer fails to *listen* to what the client wants and thereby strips them of what little control they felt they had. Now, I'm not suggesting that we should let our clients do whatever they want, whenever they want. If we did that, nothing would ever change! What I am saying is that it's important to *listen* to what they want. Our CD clients struggle to feel like they matter to anyone. "No one listens to me" is an incredibly common complaint I hear. Moreover, many individuals affected by CD are elderly, which means they're experiencing a loss of control in a whole host of domains, including their body and mind. Control over their belongings is one way they compensate, so stripping them of those belongings without their consent strips them of control and reinforces their belief that "no one listens to me."

Here's an example from one of my clients, Britt, whose well-meaning brother did exactly this.

"Don't Tell Me What to Do"

Britt

Meet Britt, a single woman in her forties who absolutely adores clothes.

When I met Britt, she was already seeing a psychologist and psychiatrist for hoarding disorder, as well as anorexia and self-diagnosed ADHD. Her mother was paying for her to see both of these professionals and agreed to pay for a professional organizing service as well, which is when Britt came into my life.

During our initial phone call, she shared that it felt like a tornado had blown through her apartment. "I feel so much shame and stigma," she told me. "I can't sleep well. I can't think. The disorganization overflows into my daily routines." These feelings are common among people affected by CD.

If Britt's tornado was made of any one thing, it was clothes. Britt prided herself on being very thrifty and loved to hunt for deals. Instead of doing laundry, she just bought more clothes. I arrived at her apartment to discover she lived in a five-hundred-square-foot ground-floor studio with her small dog, Snickers. The apartment was dark and dingy, and her entire bedroom was covered with clothes, including the floor and the bed. "Where do you sleep?" I asked. "There on the bed, on top of the clothes. I carve out a small space to lie down," she replied.

The tornado didn't stop at human clothing; it included dog clothing, as well. Britt had a new outfit for Snickers for every day of the week. She was very proud of all the outfits, many of which she had sewed herself. Yet they were mixed in with her own clothes, so when she couldn't find the outfit she wanted (which was often), she went out and bought more. It was a problem that compounded itself.

Together, Britt and I started by sorting clothes. Each piece of clothing Britt picked up from the floor she sniffed to determine whether it was clean or dirty. "Wouldn't it be safe to assume that since it's on the floor, it needs washing?" I asked.

"No" she said, "because the clean clothes are in here, too, and I don't want to wash something that's already clean."

I had only been booked for twenty-four hours of organizing, and the hours were flying by, so eventually I convinced her that we should bag up the remaining clothes—sniffed or not—and take everything to the local laundromat to be washed. That afternoon, we dropped off fifteen large garbage bags of laundry.

Britt was so territorial about her clothes, I thought she would pick them up as soon as they were ready. However, she put off picking up her laundry for so long that I finally picked it up for her. When I went inside, the attendant informed me that Britt had requested a rush job, so I now owed even more money to take the laundry away with me. Also, the attendant asked for a tip. I called Britt and asked if she'd like me to leave a tip, but she said no, that she'd come by another time and pay the tip. The attendant was displeased, and it was an uncomfortable situation, but it was a learning opportunity. This was not an arrangement I would repeat in the future.

Before helping Britt put away the bags of clean clothing, I asked some questions to check on her well-being. "Do you feel like you deserve a comfortable place to call your home?" I asked.

She replied flatly, "No." Her eyes started to well up. "It's hard for me to ask for help. I asked my mom for help, but she couldn't come. My brother came over one time to help me, but he was critical of me and just threw my clothes out without permission. He thought he was being helpful, but it was traumatic and hurtful."

Britt's clothes were a symbol of her self-worth. By casually throwing them away without her permission, her brother (unintentionally) made her feel as though he was tossing aside her feelings and deeming them unimportant. This is how it can feel to any individual affected by CD when an organizer (in Britt's case, a family member) takes over without working with the client to understand the meaning behind their belongings.

Unfortunately, I wasn't able to spend enough time with Britt to help her make meaningful adjustments in her clothing hoarding. We finished the 24-hour contract, and although her mother paid for another 24 hours of organizing, Britt canceled the service. (She actually tried to get her hands on her mother's money by asking me to refund it to her, but I refused and returned the money to her mother.) Britt clearly has more work to do around her self-worth. Sometimes, people just aren't ready to face the feelings their possessions protect.

Listening Shows Compassion

Listening is of utmost importance when it comes to showing compassion for our clients and helping them feel heard and in control. I rarely do much talking when I'm working with my clients, particularly in the beginning when I'm first forging a relationship with them. It's important for me to learn who they are, what they want, and how they operate, and I can only do that by listening. Also, I need to earn their trust, and I can do that by listening to them without judgment. How many people in their lives do that? For my clients, not many.

When I do converse, I make an effort to normalize their feelings and reactions. I relate a lot of what they're saying to my own experience, to show that I'm not perfect, either, but that there are ways to get through these feelings and experiences. Being vulnerable like this is another way to establish trust. However, I never say, "This is how I did it, so this is how you should do it, too." There is no one size fits all, and as soon as you introduce "should," you take away their control. Instead, the client and I work through different suggestions. I'll ask, "Have you thought about this?" and if they say, "I've tried that, and it won't work," I offer up a new suggestion. We keep going until we land on something they're willing to try. It might not be the solution that works best in the end, but if I can get them to try it, that is progress.

Feelings Surpass "Stuff"

The third, and perhaps most significant way cleanouts fail is that they focus on the stuff and not the person. In other words, the organizer gets distracted by the belongings and fails to address how their client *feels* about their space and about themselves. Yet without addressing this root cause, no amount of surface-level organizing will help.

Here's the emotional cycle I see most often with my clients:

The client decides they want to clean up. As they look around their home, they see piles of items taking up space all over the floor, countertops, tables, and shelves. Feelings of anxiety and despair overwhelm them as they look around their cluttered home and recognize the impact it has on their life. Stacks of dated magazines and old unopened mail are scattered about. Clothes they haven't worn in years are spilling out of their closets and drawers. This is their home—a place where they should feel comfortable and of which they should be proud. Yet when they look around, they're not proud, they're exhausted. They think to themselves, "How did I let it go so far?" Then the negative self-talk snowballs, and all of a sudden, they feel worse than when they started.

Believe it or not, what I just described are the *good* days—at least initially. These are days when a client is feeling inspired to clean up. Quickly, however, they get overwhelmed. They don't know where to start, a shortcoming for which they'll blame themselves, and soon a good day becomes a bad day. They're overwhelmed, frustrated, and tired of being tired. This cycle is nothing new, so why are they even trying? They ultimately stop struggling and settle into feeling like they don't deserve to get help or live a better life.

I've witnessed these emotions time and again with people who are affected by CD, and I will tell you: the reason the SHiFT® Method works is because it's not about a one-time cleanout; it's about taking the time to get to know the individual behind the clutter. It requires acknowledging the realness of their emotions offering hope that the emotions stopping them now won't stop them forever. They deserve to get all the help they want and need. They deserve a better life.

After a professional organizer takes the time to really listen to a client, "there seems to be a shift, a quiet exhale of relief [from my] clients, a belief that getting organized is attainable," shared Jill Yesko, author of *I'm Right Here: 10 Ways to Get Help for Hoarding and Chronic Disorganization*. That exhale, that SHiFT®, is what we're after.

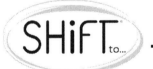

SHiFT to...

saying, "I matter, and I am more than my clutter."

When you feel anxiety and defeat begin to creep in, repeat the mantra: "I matter, and I am more than my clutter."

Getting Started

When facing a defeated, deflated client for the first time, it can be difficult to know where to begin. I'll often start by pointing out that their home didn't get this way overnight. Once clients examine the timeline that led to their life getting so cluttered, most recognize that it will take a lot of hard work to undo the accumulation of stuff and, just as importantly, work through the emotions that led to the extreme clutter. However, recognizing is not the same as doing, and there will be many moments of frustration and defeat ahead. It will take consistent reassurances from you throughout the process of decluttering that they *can* do this and it *will* be worthwhile.

Here are some other tactics I follow to help my clients (and myself!) progress on the path toward corralling their clutter and living fuller, more deserving lives.

Define Expectations

One of the most important CD organization tips I can offer is to define expectations with your client. One of the things people affected by CD struggle with is the goal of perfection. Ditch perfection at the door! No one is perfect; it's impossible to achieve. Instead, tell your client that you're actively avoiding perfection and aiming instead for "good enough." Good enough is achievable, right? And it still gets the job done!

To illustrate: When I first start working with a new client, I typically begin by asking about their pain points. I'll narrow this list down to a room where we can start decluttering, and then I'll work with them to get it into "good enough" shape. For example, if the best place to start is their bedroom, we'll declutter enough to determine which belongings are important to their daily lives and which are disruptive and can be donated or tossed. We are *not* trying to create a bedroom that looks like it came out of a catalogue; we're not even necessarily trying to get everything off the floor! My goal is to help them make the space comfortable and livable so their quality of life improves. This instills confidence in them, helps them begin to trust me, and opens the door for them to discover "wow, it feels good to live a nicer space."

Explore Feelings

To help your client create a space that is both comfortable and livable *while* ensuring that they feel heard and in control, you'll need to help them recognize their own feelings about their belongings. Here are a few questions to ask:

- How do you feel when you bring something new to the house?
- How do you feel when you're surrounded by your items?
- How would you feel about tossing things out?
- Why don't you want to toss out these items?
- Where are these feelings coming from? Where do you feel them in your body?

These aren't questions you can ask one time and move on; you'll need to ask them again and again throughout the organizing process. By frequently exploring questions like these, you bring awareness to the feelings or emotions hidden behind the items your client is protecting. There are no right or wrong answers; this exercise simply serves as a means of bringing these feelings to the forefront of their mind, so they can recognize how feelings are influencing their actions.

Find Parameters

Of course, as we agreed before, you can't let feelings continue to dictate your client's actions. That's what they've been doing all along! Therefore, you need to help them set parameters. The best way to do this is to find what parameters they've already put in place for themselves and begin to work within those parameters. You may need to be patient and pay extremely close attention to find your client's parameters, but they exist. Maybe someone keeps all of their paperwork in a single room of the house. That room may be stuffed to the gills with a mess of paper and envelopes, but it's still a parameter because it's a way they're already organizing. Therefore, it's something you can use as a reliable scaffold to build other organizing habits.

Here are a few other examples, to help you see the types of parameters your clients might set:

I had one client who bought too much stuff and then tried to hide it from her husband. One of her favorite items to buy was candles. The parameter I identified was that she wanted to store all of her candles in a particular drawer. When we measured, we found the drawer could fit only twelve candles. She owned far more than twelve candles, so we agreed that she couldn't buy any more, and she needed to whittle her current collection down to twelve.

When we began trying to prune her candle collection, she didn't want to get rid of any. When I asked her to choose her favorites, she responded, "They're all my favorite!" So, I instructed her to pick up one candle at a time, give it a sniff, pause to see how she felt about it, and describe to me why she liked (or didn't like) it. As she sniffed each candle, certain ones lit her up, and she would gush about why she liked that candle so much. We considered those to be her favorites. Once she had selected her twelve favorite candles to put in the drawer, I told her we would donate the other candles to someone else who loves candles. "They might become that other person's favorite candles," I told her. The idea that her beloved candles could bring someone else joy helped her part with them.

Another client could not bring herself to part with her child's things: drawings, awards, school tests, photos—you name it, she'd kept it. Her study was filled with mounds and mounds of sentimental papers and bric-a-brac. "I know I can't keep all this stuff, but what do I do?" she asked.

From our conversations, I determined that she was afraid of losing these special memories of her daughter. Fear was the emotion driving her actions, and memories were the parameter. Therefore, rather than push her to toss out what she felt were true emotional experiences (in the form of tangible objects), I started suggesting other ways she could preserve the memories or even make new ones. One suggestion was to take pictures of the items. (In today's cloud computing era, we can save as many photos as we want without taking up a single centimeter of physical space!)

Another suggestion was to make the sorting and pruning activity a bonding experience with her daughter. Here was how I proposed it to her: "Sit down with your daughter, pull out all the stuff, and go through it together. Laugh, recall memories, and let your daughter be the one to tell you, 'It's OK, Mom, you can get rid of that.' Or, if something has special meaning to her, set it aside to save. It's OK to keep some of this stuff, but let's contain it to a single bin." My client and her daughter have made a tradition to do this memory-sorting exercise every year, and it has been a huge step toward keeping her clutter at bay.

"You Are Not Your Things"

Here's what we're ultimately trying to get clients to understand:

You're not throwing yourself away. You're still here. You are present.

You are made up of your emotions, your memories, your health, and your relationships.

Memories reside within you, not in the items you keep. You are many things, but you are not your things.

How to Practice Feelings of Worthiness

It's easy for clients to get into the mindset that they don't deserve better because of their current situation. This is a well-trodden mental path! If they're hard on themselves every day and tell themselves they don't deserve a healthy lifestyle, they will eventually believe this to be true—the brain is *that* powerful.

However, the repeat-until-you-believe phenomenon works in reverse, too. By encouraging them to practice positive thoughts, we can help our clients create positive mindsets that change the way they value themselves. We want them to feel worthy and believe that who they are matters more than their clutter.

Of course, it's called "practice" for a reason—sometimes you have to fake it until you make it. One way to fake it is to pretend to be someone else. Ask your client to think of how their best friend speaks to them. This is how they should try to speak to themself: kindly, with compassion and encouragement.

This is also how you, their organizer, should speak with them. As you help your client organize, even if they toss out only one item that day, offer encouragement and help them give themselves positively reinforcement. Have them say out loud:

"I am proud of myself for _____ today."

"I did a good job on _____ ."

"I did well today."

If they couldn't discard or give something away that day, have them say out loud:

"I am taking things one step at a time."

"I will try again tomorrow."

"It's OK to take things slow."

As Martin Luther King, Jr. said, "If you can't fly then run, if you can't run then walk, if you can't walk then crawl, but whatever you do, you have to keep moving forward." Celebrating every win, big or small, helps make progress.

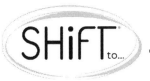

believing you are worthy.

You have always been worthy.

Whether you grew up with little or nothing at all,

Whether your parents had hoarding disorder,

Whether you developed an unhealthy attachment to things,

Whatever the situation, neither your past nor your present dictates your worth.

You are worthy of help.

You are worth the effort.

You have always been worthy of a better life.

You deserve a better life.

It's time for you to believe it.

Learning Worth and Deservingness
Marion

Meet Marion, a middle-aged woman who lives with her wife Cindy in their two-story home.

In many ways, Marion has been dealt a rough hand in life. She has been diagnosed with bipolar disorder, along with ADHD and a whole host of other health issues.

When I met Marion, initially over Zoom during the COVID-19 pandemic, her mother had recently passed away. Marion's mother was a very important person in her life. The two had been close all the way up until her death, and Marion was taking it hard. Marion's feelings were exacerbated by her conviction that her mother had been killed due to negligence by her caregivers. Marion was now not only faced with the typical barrage of financial and legal responsibilities an only child endures when their second parent passes, but she also felt responsible to pursue legal action against the caregivers. All of this pressure made Marion feel paralyzed, and the less progress she made, the more frustrated and depressed she felt.

As I worked with Marion virtually, I came to understand that while she and her mother had a loving relationship, her mother wasn't the best role model when it came to self-esteem and feeling deserving. Like most women of her generation, Marion's mother was a stay-at-home mom—a role she did not regard very highly. She was openly self-deprecating, so this is what Marion learned was "normal."

When it was finally safe for me to do so, I visited Marion in her home. By this point, Marion was spiraling. Her clutter wasn't terrible—I assessed her home as a Level II on the ICD® Clutter–Hoarding Scale®—but her partner, Cindy, was considerably neater, which was causing problems in their relationship. Cindy had claimed an office and bathroom to herself, and Marion tried to steer clear of these rooms because she was "too messy." Marion's messiness was an ongoing issue, and it had gotten to the point where Cindy was threatening to leave Marion if Marion didn't get organized.

"I promised to clean up my act," Marion told me. "But it's just gotten worse over the years, even more so after my mother was killed. Honestly, I don't know how Cindy has managed to stay with someone so fatigued who has all of these cognitive problems and a mood disorder." These were the words of someone who felt tired, defeated, and undeserving of love.

To begin our SHiFT® work, I helped Marion set goals. We started by organizing her living room. When that was accomplished, she shared her second, secret goal with me: to have a dog. She'd had a dog growing up and desperately wanted another one but felt she didn't deserve to bring a dog into her cluttered, disorganized home. If Cindy's love was already in question, she didn't want to do anything to jeopardize it more, even if getting a dog was something Marion really wanted.

As we worked together, I realized that Marion's feelings of inadequacy and unworthiness were leading her to deprioritize herself within her relationship. For example, Cindy liked peace and quiet, so Marion would play her music only when Cindy wasn't home. But Marion loved music! Whenever I came over to help her organize, she would turn on the radio and instantly became more lively and joyful. In fact, we agreed that because music gives her so much joy, she should keep her large CD collection rather than trying to pare it down.

My next step was to help Marion learn to communicate to Cindy her own needs and priorities. I reassured Marion that Cindy loves her and wants what is best for her. (After all, Cindy was paying for some of the organizing time—a clear indicator that she wanted this relationship to work!) Therefore, if music brought Marion so much joy, Cindy wouldn't want to take that away; Marion just needed to communicate its importance in her life, and they could then set up boundaries like "no music during working hours" when Cindy was at home.

Finally, when her home felt tidy enough and she had practiced communicating her needs to Cindy, Marion brought up the idea of getting a dog. To her surprise, Cindy agreed, and now Marion happily dotes on Precious, her rescue dog.

Organizing her home, her paperwork, and her storage units helped Marion feel powerful and in control of her life. Now that her kitchen is tidy, she's bought new pots and pans and resumed one of her favorite hobbies, cooking. Her relationship with Cindy grew stronger as Cindy saw the effort Marion was making, and the resulting progress gave them back their home that they could share together. Marion is learning to live a joyful, deserving life.

Collaborative Care

Of course, not every client can learn to live a deserving life with just the help of a professional organizer. In truth, most won't. We can help them make some progress, but many of our clients' needs go beyond what we can provide. This is especially true of mental health needs.

When it comes to mental health, I cannot overemphasize the importance of encouraging your client to reach out to a mental health therapist. When they're good at what they do, these professionals are worth their weight in gold. From ADHD to bipolar disorder, getting a handle on mental health disorders is a crucial step in creating the mental fortitude that can ultimately result in sustained behavior change.

The ideal scenario is a collaborative care arrangement between yourself, the therapist, and your client. Sue West, CPO-CD® and former ICD® president, emphasized that "collaborative therapy is a really positive and supportive way to help someone with a brain-based challenge to sustain success using the skills they have learned with a coach or professional organizer." In other words, therapists can help to reinforce and engrain the mindsets and skills we teach our clients.

On the flip side, many therapists see their clients in an office or virtually on a small computer or phone screen; they don't go into homes. That is why the services we, as professional organizers, offer are so crucial. We are on the front lines with the client in their own home, seeing emotions emerge in real time. In a collaborative care arrangement, we can share this valuable information with the client's therapist, helping to inform the support they provide and thereby enhancing its effectiveness.

Thought Box

" Are you willing to take steps to improve your well-being? Are you willing to make an appointment with a therapist? Are you willing to share your emotional burden with someone who cares? "

Highest Highs and Lowest Lows

Don

If you remember from Chapter 4, Don first hired me to help him handle the paperwork for businesses he'd inherited from his father. However, our relationship quickly moved beyond that need, as his CD was affecting many other areas of his life.

I worked with Don for several years, and it took until our second year of working together for him to share that when he was a child, his father had continually belittled and verbally abused him. This had not changed with time; even as an adult, he endured harsh criticism from his father and, as a result, often felt he was never good enough. He also shared that his ex-wife had physically beaten him and left him with a fractured skull and a TBI that he has been forced to manage ever since.

Depressed and defeated, Don was not caring for himself. He was not eating nutritious food or exercising. At one point, Don hired a personal trainer at a local gym. He prepaid $5,000 for fifty sessions, with the goal of losing weight. He went once. Unfortunately, having the financial resources and hiring an accountability partner weren't enough for Don to fulfill this goal.

The longer I worked with Don, the further I saw his mental and physical health deteriorate. He continued to gain weight, began to self-medicate, and eventually turned to illicit drug use. I knew Don needed to see a mental health therapist, and I tried over and over to convince him to make an appointment, but he never did.

Eventually, I had to stop working with Don. The possibility of making a SHiFT® had moved too out of reach. Don couldn't hear the message of "i" (I am deserving) or "H" (health) in the SHiFT® Method; his physical and mental health needs were too severe.

This is the final text I sent to Don, to end our relationship.

Happy Thursday Don!

I know you have a lot going on and are overwhelmed. I would love for you to make yourself a priority. That means you must put yourself first. Begin seeing a therapist, drug rehabilitation, see a doctor for the narcolepsy and eat healthy. It all matters. You are worth it and you matter! Because it's critical that you get help, I feel we need to pause organizing services until you are strong enough to work together.

Don, you are such a great person, and you need to put yourself first. What I see now is someone who is self-destructing and that scares me. If you don't put yourself first your life could be in danger.

When you recognize you are important and get help and are back on your feet, I will be there to support you. Until then, I am pausing our relationship. I am refunding $1540, which represents today, 12/16, less the cancellation fee + the next session on 12/21. You have no more scheduled sessions.

Wishing you strength and sending healthy boundaries.

Jen

Despite his financial resources and hiring me as an accountability partner, Don needed help I could not provide. As organizers, we need to recognize and respond to these unfortunate situations. As much as we may want to help someone, there eventually comes a time when we need to step away for our own health and safety. For me, while it broke my heart, this was one of those times.

Don died less than three weeks later.

Learning to Live a Deserving Life
Hank

To end on a happier note, let's return to one of my all-time favorite client success stories: Hank.

At the start of our work together, Hank absolutely did not feel deserving. He was neglecting his social relationships (he no longer hosted friends or family in his home), his health (bathing in the sink, breathing in decades of dust), and more. Early on, he shared that he felt like he'd never fit in anywhere, and the dissolution of his marriage only reinforced that belief. He no longer even believed he was worth the time of his daughter, who was the one who had hired me to help her dad.

Yet a tiny flame of hope still burned inside Hank. I know this because with time, persistence, and a whole lot of work, Hank made the SHiFT®. As I cleaned and tidied each room of his house with him, he gained another foothold in feeling heard, in control, and deserving of a nicer living space. Our work progressed to the point that Hank was willing (begrudging, nervous, but willing) to *move out of his home* so it could be renovated. This is so rare that no other professional organizer I've ever met has had a hoarding client consent to this. And yet Hank managed to do it, because he finally felt worthy of not only a decent living space, but also of hosting his family again in his own home.

In the time I worked with Hank, he transformed from a withdrawn, stubborn recluse to a gregarious, generous father and grandfather. And really, the person who emerged was Hank's true self—the person he'd been, inside, the entire time. He just needed to climb out from underneath all that clutter and realize that he was deserving of family, love, and happiness. He needed to feel worthy, and now he does.

Conclusion

Mental and emotional well-being are at the core of the SHiFT® Method. For our clients, this comes down to self-esteem; self-worth; and feeling heard, in control, and deserving of a full, happy life.

When they begin their organizing journey with us, or even when they're several steps along that path, most clients probably won't genuinely *feel* "I am deserving." That's OK. Our work happens incrementally, through consistent reinforcement, until the client naturally begins to tell themselves what we have been telling them all along: you are more than your belongings. You can do this because you are worth it.

How did Britt, Marion, Hank, and Don use the "i" in SHiFT® to learn how to live a full, deserving life?

Britt

- Made decisions that strengthened her self-confidence
- Started washing her clothes once a week after work, which enabled her to spend time with friends on the weekends
- Improved her relationship with her mom, at least temporarily

Marion

- Learned to put her own needs on par with the needs of others
- Adopted a dog, Precious, which she'd always wanted to do
- Negotiated with her partner, Cindy, times when Marion could play music in their house

Hank

- Moved out of his dilapidated home to allow it to be renovated
- Stood up for his own desires and preferences during the renovation (for instance, specifying the floor tiles he wanted and his favorite paint color, yellow)
- Invited his family over for meals and weekend visits

Don

- Don was deserving, just as every human is. Unfortunately, he couldn't see it. Sometimes, clients aren't yet ready or able to change their self-beliefs. All we can do is try our best to help them and patiently await the day they decide "I am worth it."

Think, Write...Deserve

1. Describe what a deserving life looks like for you.

2. Negative self-talk derails your desire to live a deserving life. What steps are you taking to negate negative self-talk?

3. Positive self-talk sets you on the path to living a deserving life. What are some things you can say to yourself that will feel encouraging and uplifting?

4. You put your family, pets, and work first. Imagine putting yourself first. What does that look like? In what ways does putting yourself first better support the life you want?

5. How are you going to change your narrative so you are deserving and worthy?

Chapter 6

"F" is for Finances

SHiFT

"When you understand that your self-worth is not determined by your net worth, then you'll have financial freedom."

—Suze Orman

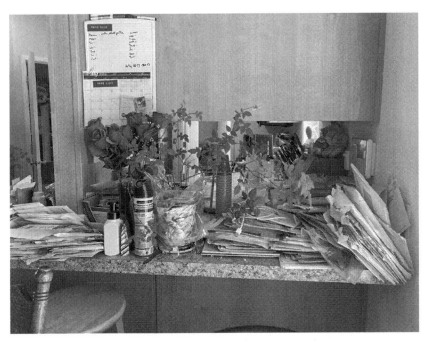

Photo credit: Connie Anderson

Postponed decisions and a delay in processing mail add up.

Finally we have reached the dreaded "F": Finances. With the exception of day traders and certain hobbyist investors, I've met almost no one who thinks of money fondly. Sure, receiving money feels great, but managing money? Making sure you have enough to live your life now and in the future? Paying bills, owing taxes, and simply deciding the best places to spend your hard-earned income? It's stressful.

Few of us, including our clients, have any formal financial education. We've done the best we can by mimicking our parents, listening to our friends, and absorbing ideas from society at large. Some of us were blessed with an upbringing, personality traits, or even just intuitive sense that's made managing our money easier. Unfortunately, people with CD experience the opposite— their tendencies toward clutter and hoarding make it extremely challenging to stay on top of their finances.

Some clients will admit they have a distorted relationship with money. One client told me, "I just don't want to think about it [money]—it makes me sick. I have a vague idea of what I am spending, but I don't want to confront it." Another client described her tendency to overspend as a shame cycle: "Spending money to fill an emotional need creates a shame cycle. Buyer's remorse may ring a bell."

Other clients, however, cannot see how CD has contributed to their financial woes. "I'm a cheapskate!" they'll announce, yet they are surrounded by so much stuff that they are forced to carve out pathways to move from room to room. I had a client proudly tell me she regularly drives thirty minutes each way to cash in a few bags of recyclable bottles at the five-cent beverage container deposit. She receives six dollars for her bounty! Yet while it was positive for her to get those bottles out of her house, her financial motivation was flawed. She never considered that her time plus the cost of gasoline entirely offset her six-dollar reward; cashing in those bottles was, in fact, *costing* her money.

In this chapter, we're going to review the primary ways CD can lead our clients into financial chaos, and I'll offer some of the solutions that I've developed. Before I begin, however, I want to emphasize that I am not a financial planner, accountant, CPA, or any other type of financial expert. I am a woman with a variety of life experiences who owns a successful business and has helped dozens of clients affected by CD get back on their feet. All the ideas I present are based on my experiences and the experiences of my clients. I hope they will help you develop some strategies of your own!

How Chronic Disorganization Leads to Over-spending

Let's quickly review some common characteristics of people who experience CD. According to the Institute of Challenging Disorganization®, these include:

- Live in a cluttered space
- Are unable to quickly find their things

- Get distracted easily
- Have a hard time letting things go
- Keep a large number of items that aren't seen as a need

It may not be immediately apparent, but these characteristics impact not only how people affected by CD live their daily lives, but also how they manage (or mismanage) their money. Let's start by grouping some characteristics:

Living in a cluttered space + unable to find their things (including bills that need to be paid!) + getting distracted easily

When someone is surrounded by clutter, they're going to have trouble finding their belongings when they need them. This issue is compounded when that person is easily distracted—a characteristic that especially affects clients who have ADHD. Oftentimes, they'll intend to put an item back where it belongs, get distracted, lay it down somewhere else, and then deem it "missing" the next time they need it.

The result? If it's a physical item, they go out and buy another one. If it's a bill, they accrue a late fee.

Having a hard time letting things go + keeping a large number of items that aren't needed

Every client affected by CD saves items they don't need, although the reasons behind this behavior vary. While some clients save items for more sentimental reasons (discussed in Chapter 5), some actually have well-intentioned financial motivations. I've worked with many clients who believe that "hoarding" everything will save them money in the future. Someday down the line, they reason, they'll need the item and will have it readily available. And some items, like antiques, might increase in value! This may be true for some of their belongings, but the reality is that it's not true for most, and it's definitely not true of *everything* they own. By saving everything, the person often ends up spending even more money than they would have "saved" in the first place—either on storage units to hold the items or on house repairs (because, as you will see, or may have already experienced, clutter can lead to serious structural damage in a house or apartment).

In the remainder of this chapter, we're going to cover what I've found to be the main contributors to financial disarray in my clients' lives. These are:

- Buying duplicates
- Falling prey to marketing and "sales"
- Avoiding mail (and therefore bills)
- Spending on storage units
- Allowing clutter to degrade the integrity of their home

No matter which contributors you are facing, there is a tactic you must implement at the outset of working with your client. It won't be easy for them, but it's essential. When I work with someone who has a spending issue, I tell them that in order to work with me, they must stop making any nonessential purchases until we get their finances under control. That means they are only permitted to buy things like food, toilet paper, and gas; items like clothes, shoes, decorations, and games are not allowed. That is the deal. They must promise, and they must follow through, or we cannot work together.

With that agreement in place, let's get going!

Duplicates

When you can't find an item, what do you do? You buy a new one, of course. For those of us without CD, this occasionally results in buying a duplicate of something we didn't need. Who hasn't bought a new tube of toothpaste, only to find an unopened tube in the medicine cabinet at home?

Individuals affected by CD, however, often buy the same items repeatedly because they can *never* find what they're looking for at home. Nail clippers, measuring spoons, reading glasses, scissors . . . "they must be hidden somewhere!" And they are: these items are hidden amid the clutter, where our client cannot find them. Instead of going through the hassle of trying to look for what they want, the client goes out and buys the item anew. In the short term, this solution is easier, but those constant duplicate purchases add up, both in terms of money spent *and* in terms of added clutter.

If you remember Don's story from Chapter 4, he had amassed more over-the-counter medicines and first aid supplies than a person could ever use in one lifetime. (It's impossible to imagine a scenario where someone would need twenty-five tubes of Neosporin!) Yet because he constantly misplaced the supplies he had—at least until we devised a solution—he kept ordering more, leading him to spend money he didn't have on items he would never use.

Solution 1: The Moratorium

In many cases, the moratorium I put on my client's extraneous purchases at the outset of our work together helps put them on the path toward solving this "duplicates" problem. During the time when they're forbidden from buying yet another pack of scrapbooking stickers, we'll be organizing their craft room, and, lo and behold, we'll find sixteen packs of stickers! Then, once we've established a system to keep the craft room organized, they are able to find their stickers and no longer need to buy any until their stash runs low.

Solution 2: End Auto-Buy and "Subscriptions"

For Don, in addition to being unable to find his first aid materials amid his cluttered house, a big contributor to his perpetual first aid purchases was his Amazon Prime account. When he started ordering supplies online, he loved the idea of saving 5 percent and therefore chose the "subscribe" option. However, saving 5 percent on items you don't need and never use isn't *saving* any money at all; it's wasting one hundred percent of the money you spent!

When I'd amassed all of Don's supplies and shown him that he didn't need more, I sat down with him at his computer and clicked "unsubscribe" on each item in his Amazon subscription list. The thing to note is that I had to physically do this with him.

I didn't give Don instructions and leave him to his own devices; I sat beside him for every mouse click. This is often the extent to which you'll need to help a client make changes in their financial life. Change is scary! But with us by their side offering reassurance and encouragement, it's possible.

"Sales"

10% off! 50% off! Limited-time offer. Buy one get one FREE!

Does your pulse quicken at the sight of these ads? Mine does. I suspect most people get a little rush at the thought of a good deal. Shopping triggers the release of the feel-good neurotransmitter dopamine, and snagging something on sale feels even better.

Companies know this. It's why they have sales, and it's why their marketing teams promote said sales relentlessly. When a consumer is feeling good and focusing on the money they're "saving," they buy more and spend more. This keeps capitalism alive and well.

We're all affected by these tactics, but to varying degrees. If the average person's vulnerability to the allure of shopping and "sales" is around a level 6, I'd put the vulnerability of someone affected by CD at a level 9, and probably more realistically a level 10! The reason is threefold. First, my clients almost always believe what the companies tell them. "Buy this now so you don't miss out" makes it sound like the company is looking out for them, the consumer. You and I know that's not true, but many clients are naive; they genuinely believe the company is looking out for their best interests. Oftentimes, they view companies as experts, and they're always on the lookout for an expert. (Fortunately, this plays to our advantage as professional organizers—we're experts, too!)

Second, people affected by CD experience extremely acute FOMO (fear of missing out). When they see a sale or other limited-time offer, they worry that it won't happen again and that if they don't buy the thing right now, that price will be gone forever. The same thing goes for unique items: my client Barbara would regularly browse eBay, and when she saw something that was one of a kind, she "had to have it"—even if it just stayed in its box in her storage unit. She was too afraid of missing out!

Third, reacting to sales is a form of distraction. When you're rushing to nab a great deal, you don't have to think about who you are, what you really want, or your ultimate purpose in life. Put another way, when people are distracted, they don't have to face reality. Many of our clients are living a reality that is dire, so it's no surprise that they're seeking distractions. Unfortunately, the more they buy, the worse their reality gets.

Solution 1: Explain, Repeat, Remind

The most important thing we can do for clients who are "sales addicts" is help them understand what's actually behind the marketing messages they receive. My main take-home message is: it's all about money. Marketers are paid to deceive and to create urgency to buy their product. Most times, it's not even a product anyone needs!

Here's an exercise I do with clients when they're eyeing a marketing flier or social media ad: I ask, "Pretend this wasn't on sale. Would you still buy it?" Ninety percent of the time they say "no." Before they can squeeze in a "but," I add, "If you save 50 percent, you still pay 50 percent. How much do you save if you don't buy it at all?" Sometimes I have to use dollars and cents to illustrate the point, but eventually they get it.

Now, let's say the client claims they'd buy the item even if it weren't on sale. Then I ask, "Okay, but if you were buying it full price, would you buy it *right now*?" The answer is almost always "no," at which point I reassure them that sales almost always come back around. The feeling of urgency they're experiencing is real, but the urgency itself is not. It's okay to let this opportunity pass!

These types of conversations, where I try to educate my clients and also reassure them, are constant and ongoing. This sort of SHiFT® in thinking takes time. Ultimately, my goal is to help them understand that they're just a commodity to companies, and they should learn to trust themselves over these false "experts." If they do, they will ultimately spend their time, energy, and even hard-earned money on fostering real relationships with family and friends, and they'll be happier for it.

Solution 2: Boost Their Confidence

As you're educating your clients and reassuring them, help them practice making wise purchasing decisions. Don't just offer a list of dos and don'ts; get them to think through situations and come to their own conclusion. The goal here is to boost their confidence and help them learn to trust themselves. They don't always need an "expert" to tell them what to do; they can decide on their own!

Fooled by Marketing
Skylar

As you may remember from Chapter 3, Skylar was a landscape architect who hired me as a last-ditch effort to save her business from crumbling. Her business operations were best described by Ari Tuchman, in his book *More Attention, Less Deficit Success Strategies for Adults with ADHD,* as "float[ing] through life from crisis to crisis, living two steps in front of the avalanche—and sometimes two steps behind it." When I arrived, she was essentially buried.

Part of what buried Skylar's business was her vulnerability to marketing. She regularly received emails and direct marketing advertisements encouraging her to get certified in this thing or get listed in that directory. Instead of evaluating the value such certifications and directory listings would add to her business (would she actually gain more clients, and would they really pay higher rates?), she fell prey to the "act now" urgency and seeming "expert" guidance and signed up for every one. These credentials, memberships, and listings required regular ongoing payments, so the more she accumulated, the higher her overhead rose.

When I came in to help Skylar get her finances under control, I immediately assessed which memberships and credentials were costing money without bringing in any revenue, and we canceled them. I also convinced her to fire her bookkeeper, who was overcharging while underdelivering—another case of misplaced trust in someone who *should* have been an expert.

Unfortunately for Skylar, all of these efforts were too little, too late. She owed everyone, from the IRS to her own employees, and she couldn't come up with the money. Ultimately, she filed for bankruptcy and left town. While that was the end of our work together, I am hopeful some of what we did taught her to be more prudent about the people and organizations she chooses to trust with her money.

Mail

If I were to point to one issue my CD clients face across the board—men, women, young, old, rich, poor—it's mail. There's not a client home I've encountered that wasn't filled with an abundance of mail. And after many, many conversations, I've determined that the reason mail is a problem for people affected by CD boils down to two underlying causes: uncertainty and fear.

Uncertainty is a recurring theme when it comes to how CD affects a person's finances. In the case of purchases, it causes our clients to seek out "experts" and fall prey to advertising campaigns that seem to demonstrate expertise. When it comes to mail, uncertainty creates a sort of paralysis. Our clients aren't stupid; they know that junk mail should go straight into the recycle bin. They just don't trust themselves to properly evaluate whether a certain piece of mail is important or not, so they resort to saving all of it "just in case."

This "just in case" mentality dovetails into the other contributing factor: fear. Saving everything "just in case" comes from a combination of uncertainty about what to do with it and fear that what they choose to do with it will be wrong. For instance, if they accidentally throw out a bill, that's going to create problems down the line. However, they're often equally afraid they'll throw out a flier about a sale they believe they'd regret missing. That's how it all ends up in piles throughout the house, with birthday cards mixed in with bills, catalogues, political mailers, and goodness knows what else.

There's also another type of fear that anyone who has been financially strapped has felt: fear of the unmarked white envelope. These types of envelopes often contain bills, collection notices, or other financially unpleasant news. It takes a certain degree of resolve to open these envelopes and face one's financial reality, and many of our clients are masters at avoiding unpleasant realities. Therefore, they simply don't open the envelope. Some might tell themselves "I'll get to it later," but they never do. Eventually they forget about it, and it gets lost in the clutter. They've sidestepped a few moments of discomfort; yet the more of these envelopes they avoid, the higher the late fees climb, and the worse their finances become.

Solution 1: Educate and Organize

Sometimes, the solution to a client's mail avoidance is as simple as educating them about what counts as important and what does not. This worked with one of my clients who had autism: we sat down together at each session and examined the mail that had arrived. I started out asking him to identify different pieces of mail and the intentions the sender may have had.

"What is this?" (It's a flyer.)

"What's a flyer?" (A flyer is a piece of mail that typically has all of its writing on the exterior, as opposed to the writing being inside an envelope. Often it is very colorful, with big flashy font and images.)

"Who is sending it to you, and what are they trying to accomplish?" (A department store wants you to visit their store and spend money.)

"Now that you recognize what this piece of mail is, is it worth spending the time to examine it closely?" (Nope, I don't need anything from that department store.)

"If you don't need this piece of mail, what do you do with it?" (Put it in the recycling bin!)

The more we repeated this exercise, the better my client got at distinguishing important mail from junk mail. For the items that were deemed important to keep, I made a mail binder and divided it into relevant categories. The purpose of mail binders is to force clients to identify exactly what the item of mail is and to then store those items in a place they can find again when they need them. I'll often include other important information in the binder, too, like passwords, emergency contact information, and job documents.

Now, you might be wondering: what about sentimental items? After all, it might seem a bit heartless to throw away a birthday card from your best friend or a thank-you note from your nephew. My rule of thumb is to have the client evaluate the item based on the amount of personalization the sender added. If it's a standard birthday card simply signed "Love, Mom and Dad," I encourage my client to toss it. After all, when will they look at it again? Probably never. If, however, the card has personal inscriptions and feels emotionally significant, it's fine to keep it. I advise stowing items like this in a memorabilia box. The client can return to the box whenever they like, and when the box gets overfull, that's an indicator that it's time to sort through the items and get rid of any that no longer feel meaningful.

Solution 2: Embrace Autopay

When it comes to paying essential bills, encourage your clients to sign up for online autopay. This helps to cut down on the mail they'll receive, which in turn cuts down on the amount of work they have to do sorting it. (Plus, it eliminates paper waste—one small contribution to preserving the environment. And I strongly believe that every contribution counts!) Autopay also eliminates the chances of missing a bill and accruing late fees or worse. Finally, it entirely circumvents that fearful unmarked-white-envelope moment and the discomfort of writing out a check and watching the account balance go down.

Now, not every client will be willing to sign up for online autopay. Even after you explain the benefits of doing it (and drawbacks of not), some clients are so fearful of the internet, they will simply refuse. In these cases, simply go back to the binder method I described and develop a system for sitting down to *pay* the bills being filed away in there. This may mean creating a schedule for the client to sit down with their checkbook on the first Saturday of the month, or it may mean they pay a bill as soon as they put it into the binder. You'll have to collaborate with the client to figure out what works best for them, but no matter what, they need a system that will keep them on top of important payments.

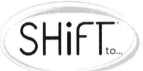

SHiFT to...

making auto-payments online.

Automatic payments can help you reduce paper clutter, pay bills on time, and avoid late fees and discontinued services.

Taking Back Financial Control
Gretchen & Graham

As shared by Connie Anderson

Meet Gretchen, a suburban wife and mother to one young daughter. Gretchen had always struggled mildly with CD, but she probably would never have reached out to me had she not lost her job. When she was fired from her banking job, Gretchen stopped opening the mail for weeks at a time. The loss of income put financial strain on her family, and this was not something she wanted to face. The longer she went without managing her mail, the worse the situation became. She and her husband, Graham, started to carry high balances on several credit cards to make ends meet. Unpaid bills began to mount. All of this created even more anxiety about processing the mail because neither Gretchen nor Graham wanted to face the collection notices, late notices, and bad credit score alerts.

Meanwhile, Graham worked a full-time job during the week and ran a side business on weekends and evenings. The problem was that Graham, while good at what he did for his side business, was a terrible accountant. By the time I arrived on the scene, Graham and Gretchen's misguided attempts at filing, invoicing clients, and tracking necessary operating permits had completely overwhelmed the couple. As a result, they had tens of thousands of dollars in uncollected revenue and virtually no billing records. The financial strain from this and from Gretchen's lack of employment were palpable and was straining the couple's marriage.

Ultimately, Gretchen and Graham filed for bankruptcy. However, they knew they needed to do better—and that's where I came in. Over six years, I worked with them to set up systems for simple tasks, like sorting mail, and complex ones, like managing Graham's side business.

It took Gretchen and Graham years to pay down their debts, and, as part of the bankruptcy terms, they had to stop using credit cards. To their surprise, this credit card freeze turned out to be a blessing in disguise. Being forced to use cash taught them how to live within their means. A year after being released from the constraints of bankruptcy, they celebrated by bringing a dog into the family, which their daughter had wanted for years. The dog they chose cost $5,000, but they could afford it because I had taught them to save money for unexpected expenses and larger-ticket purchases. From their experience with bankruptcy and their work with me, Gretchen and Graham learned a valuable lesson: by looking at their finances head-on, saving for what they wanted, and paying cash, they could avoid going back into debt.

Storage Units

When the homes of people affected by CD reach their storage capacity, with every room and closet crammed floor to ceiling, these individuals start to look elsewhere for places to put their belongings. First, they shuffle stuff from one room to another or into closets, attics, and basements. When they are out of space at home, they turn to off-site storage units. Of course, renting storage units costs money, so now our clients are not only spending money *buying* things, they are also spending money *storing* them.

Storage units range from $100 to $1,200 or more per month, depending on size. A 10' x 20' storage unit can cost up to $14,000 a year. To make matters worse, one storage unit often turns into two, then three, then four. . . . My clients have had as many as thirteen storage units, and they rent them for years. Many of my clients, when asked, can't say how long they've rented their storage units. Moreover, they have no idea how much the units are costing them. This is in part because, unlike their other bills, these clients pay for storage units using autopay. They've elected to have the fees billed straight to their credit card each month because if they fall behind, even once, their units—and all of the possessions inside—can be confiscated by the rental company.

When it comes to renting storage units, our clients are not so different from the average American; about one in eleven Americans pays to put their excess things behind a metal door, creating a self-storage industry worth $38 billion. This doesn't happen by accident—it's because of the consumerism rampant in our culture, to which our clients are especially vulnerable. What's noteworthy is that our clients are *not* the average American; their clutter is ruining their quality of life. This is why it's so important to help them move away from paying for storage units, so they can spend their money on things that make a meaningful difference in their lives.

Solution 1: Show Them the Cost

Instead of helping to fund this multi-billion-dollar industry, I encourage my clients to seriously reconsider the need for renting a storage unit and to weigh that need against the monetary costs. To do this, I show them what it's costing them to store their belongings.

First, I have them write down on a piece of paper how long they've had the storage unit (even if it's a guess) and how much they pay (per month, per year—whatever they can provide). Then, using a calculator (often on my phone), we add up how much total money they've spent on that unit. When they see the figure, they're often flabbergasted. How could they be spending so much money and not even know it? This is my opening to persuade them to *stop* needlessly spending so much money and to consolidate or eliminate their costly storage units.

Solution 2: Help Them Envision an Alternative

When cost alone isn't enough to persuade a client to relinquish their storage units, the next tactic is to help them imagine what they might be able to do with all that money. Is there an experience or activity that would make them happier but that they can't afford because their money is being sucked into storage fees? Is there someone they'd like to spend more money on? Could they improve the quality of their life, if only they had that money available? When we play this "what if" game, clients are slowly able to envision alternative futures where they are living a happier, more fulfilling life. Eventually, with gentle prodding, many can be encouraged to take the leap to get rid of at least one storage unit and try using that money in other ways.

Thought Box

66

What is the monetary, time, and energy cost of keeping and storing your belongings?

99

"Downsizing" Storage Units
Barbara

Back in Chapter 3, I briefly described helping Barbara empty out her storage units. Here is the full story of how that happened:

When I started working with her, Barbara owned not one, not two, but seven storage units. She had one ground-level unit measuring 10' x 20' and five additional units on the second level measuring 7' x 10' each. Barbara wasn't sure how long she'd been paying rent on these units, but she estimated at least fifteen years. Using simple arithmetic, I calculated she had spent over $380,000 on storage unit rental fees. When she saw the total, she quite literally couldn't believe it.

Given that the ground-floor unit was the largest and most expensive—$1,200/month—we started there. The unit was filled from floor to ceiling with meticulously labeled boxes. Barbara had been collecting and storing baking supplies for years, and in her mind, when she decided to liquidate the contents of the unit, she would sell the items and recoup some money. However, the value of the baking supplies couldn't come close to matching the years of rental fees for the unit, which is why we needed to liquidate the contents as soon as possible.

Sorting and emptying the unit took us months. One of the first things I did was reach out to a friend who owned a nearby baking supply store. My friend scheduled a "field trip" to the storage unit with the local Cake Club, so they could buy some of Barbara's stock. To prepare for the sale, Barbara and I categorized everything and hung signs to indicate the items' prices. Almost everything was new, still in its original packaging, and the Cake Club ended up buying a good deal of Barbara's baking supplies—Bundt cake pans, doilies, drying racks, cookie cutters, and more.

After the sale Barbara rented a van to finish emptying the unit. She sold vanfuls of baking supplies at cake shows, but ultimately some items needed to be donated, and other items simply got tossed. All in all, she got back only a fraction of the money that she'd spent on the items, never mind what she had spent on storage fees. If Barbara had cut her losses fifteen years ago, she would have "made" more money by closing down the storage unit and donating everything.

After we cleared out the largest unit, Barbara and I proceeded upstairs to the six other units. The task at hand was to empty and free up as many of the units as we could. We used the app Airtable to take inventory of all the items and to sort them into "sell," "keep," "donate," and "discard" categories. The Airtable data also helped Barbara to see what she already owned, thereby preventing additional (duplicate!) purchases.

In the end, Barbara wasn't able to clear out all of the remaining six units. I encouraged her to donate the contents that remained, or to have an estate sale, but at some point she got stuck emotionally and couldn't proceed. The good news is that compared to what she had been spending previously, Barbara was paying considerably less on storage unit rental fees. The bad news is that, in another fifteen years, she'll have thrown away thousands more dollars. The reality is that in most cases, we can't entirely transform our clients' thinking or decision-making—but some progress is always better than none.

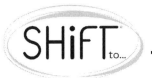

Home Damage

The final way clutter can cause financial strife is through home damage. Now, clutter itself does not necessarily "damage" a home—although it can! I once had a client who packed his apartment so full, it presented a danger to his downstairs neighbors because the structure of the building wasn't designed to support the weight of all his belongings. Scary stuff!

More often, however, homes become structurally damaged due to neglect that is perpetuated by the clutter. For example, both Barbara and Don had issues with condensation leaking from their air conditioners. Not only were they unaware of the leak because they couldn't see their air conditioners through the cluttered rooms, but even if they'd known about the leak, Don in particular could never have maneuvered through all of his belongings to actually reach the air conditioner and fix it. In both cases, the condensation leaked through the floor into the rooms below, causing mold to grow and creating costly damage. Barbara even ended up owing $40,000 to renovate and repair the damage to her downstairs neighbor's apartment!

An even more extreme example is Hank, who had to move out of his house entirely in order for it to be fully renovated. Fortunately, Hank was wealthy enough to afford such a renovation (and the months of relocating to another residence while the renovation happened), but most clients are not. And even if someone has the money, home renovations are a substantial expense that negatively impacts a person's finances and are better off avoided whenever possible.

Solution 1: Increase Awareness

People affected by CD are often unable to see beyond their stuff, both literally and figuratively. They are so engaged with their "things" that they don't think about the walls, counters, shelves, and floors supporting those things. Therefore, step one is to simply make your clients more aware of the spaces in which they are living. Once I've gotten clients to recognize the physical structures, I move toward making them aware of how their belongings are impacting those structures. They key is to start simple. Even if there is serious structural damage (or if I suspect it), I'll often start with more obvious instances of clutter-related damage: "Why did that shelf break?" "How did that door come unhinged?" This line of questioning and attention-directing is a form of education—it guides clients to their own conclusions, which is often more effective than simply telling them what happened and why. By thinking about the questions, the client is learning how their choices impact their living space and how different choices might yield better results.

Solution 2: Present Consequences

While serious damage is sometimes already done by the time I arrive, there are also many cases where the damage is minimal and can be mitigated through immediate action. In these cases, my goal is to show clients that an ounce of prevention is worth a pound of cure. Let's consider Barbara's and Don's leaky air conditioners. In these cases, if I arrived early in the "life" of the leak, I might try getting them to see and feel what is happening ("Do you see this mold? Can you feel the floorboard softening? The leak is causing that") and then follow up with what is likely to happen if the issue remains untreated ("Your ceiling could collapse, which will damage both your house and your belongings in this room and the room below"). People with CD don't always find anticipated financial repercussions to be persuasive (e.g., the cheaper immediate cost of repairing the air conditioner vs. the later more expensive cost of repairing a floor/ceiling), so I try to come up with other ways to frame the issue that will resonate more deeply. These might include safety ("The ceiling could fall on you or your loved ones") or health ("If you keep breathing in mold spores, you could develop chronic respiratory infections"). When you've worked with a client long enough, you'll understand what motivates them. Use that to your advantage!

Avoiding a Second Home Renovation

Fiona

As shared by Connie Anderson

If you remember Fiona from Chapter 4, you'll recall that I was introduced to her by her fiduciary. Fiona owned a one-bedroom apartment and, with the fiduciary's assistance, had previously renovated it after it had fallen into squalor. Now, the fiduciary was concerned the apartment was headed back to being hoarded.

When I stepped foot in Fiona's apartment for the first time, I was confronted with the overpowering stench of dirty cat litter. I found the kitchen infested with insects, and I could barely see the decrepit state of the living room because the home lacked any functional lighting. The bathroom was covered in a gray grimy filth, dirty laundry was piled high, and her turtle's tank had clearly been neglected for quite a while.

I worked with Fiona for several sessions until she stopped scheduling appointments. She claimed her finances were tied up after purchasing a sofa, but her failure to ever invite me back suggests that was merely an excuse. I remain hopeful that with the continued help of her therapist, Fiona will succeed at maintaining the weekly schedule I created to help her gain confidence and develop life skills to keep her apartment livable. If she fails, chances are that her hoarding and neglect of home maintenance will lead to another expensive home renovation.

Conclusion

The social, health-related, and self-esteem costs of CD are high—and the financial costs are, perhaps, even higher. As a professional organizer, I see three general patterns in the way my clients interact with money: ignorance, avoidance, and denial. Many clients fail to recognize their own patterns of overspending, whether on duplicates or "sales." Nearly all of them demonstrate some form of ignorance, avoidance, or denial of mounting debt in the way they treat (or, more accurately, neglect) mail. They rarely know or will willingly face the amount of money they are losing to storage unit rental fees, and few can responsibly respond, on their own, to the revelation that their disorganization is degrading the integrity of their physical home.

This is where it's our responsibility as professional organizers to provide a combination of encouragement, education, and tough love. No one wants to see a client lose their home or other valuable assets due to financial ruin. Therefore, from day one we need to be setting up schedules and structures to help our clients form better thought patterns and behaviors around money. Sometimes, this requires a cold dose of realism. Cassandra Aarssen, a professional organizer and founder of ClutterBug Organizing Services, shared a quote that I repeat often to my clients: "Remember that the money you spent on your item is gone. You are not any richer because you store this item in your home, and you won't be poorer if you let it go."

How did Skylar, Gretchen and Graham, Barbara, and Fiona use the "F" in SHiFT® to learn how to live a full, deserving life?

Skylar

- Stopped paying for certifications, listings, and services that were either overpriced or not bringing in enough revenue to justify their cost
- Learned to simplify her life by becoming an employee rather than an employer

Gretchen & Graham

- Processed mail to address financial matters—even scary ones—in a timely manner
- Paid cash in order to learn to stay within their budget
- Saved for big-ticket items they really wanted instead of spending frivolously on purchases they didn't value as much

Barbara

- Closed down her largest and most expensive storage unit, saving $14,400 a year
- Sold baking supplies to recoup some of the cost of those purchases, plus the rental unit fees

Fiona

- Recognized and admitted needing the help of a fiduciary
- Trusted in the investment of hiring professional organizers

Think, Write...Deserve

1. Are your short- and long-term goals compatible with your disposable income?

2. While spending money on things you want right now feels good, how can you get that same feeling from saving money?

3. In what ways can you break the pattern of mail avoidance?

4. Working past your fear of internet-based banking services will allow you to pay your bills on time. A friend, family, or professional organizer is willing to help you learn and set this up. If you are willing to take this step, how would paying your bills on time change your quality of life?

5. What would you do with the money you could save if you gave up paying rent on a storage unit(s)?

Chapter 7

"T" is for Time

SHifT®

"Time is finite. We don't really manage time; we manage our activities within the time we have."

—Joseph R. Ferrari, PhD

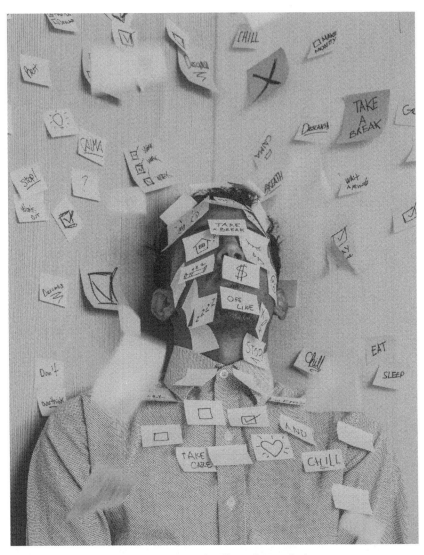

Photo Credit: Luis Villasmil, Unsplash

Too many unfinished task lists can be paralyzing.

I was once interviewed by a therapist who treats people with hoarding disorder and CD. One of the questions she asked me was, "What is your greatest challenge working with people who hoard or are chronically disorganized?" I thought long and hard about this question. There are a number of challenges! Ultimately, I told her that the issue my clients face that influences all other aspects of their CD has to do with time. My clients live primarily in the past, sometimes the future, but *never in the present*. I've heard nearly every client say some version of:

"Things are not the way they used to be."

"Someday I might need this."

"It will come in handy someday."

"It may not work, but I will fix it someday."

What my clients don't say is, "I am really comfortable with how things are right now. I realize time is precious, and I want to make the most of it."

Ultimately, being stuck in the past or perpetually looking ahead to the future means that my clients—and probably your clients, too—are squandering time in the present. Consider this scenario, which I hear from many clients:

Suddenly it's 9:00 p.m., and the well-intended "to do" list for the day is still incomplete. They had started sorting mail, but then they worried they might want all of these flyers tomorrow or next week or the next time they go shopping. So they moved on to scheduling a lunch with a friend, but then they remembered something embarrassing they said the last time they were with the friend, so they put off finishing that task, too. One thing led to another, and before they knew it, the day was coming to a close.

It happens. But what if it happens every day? The result is missing important deadlines and appointments and failing to meet personal goals. Their *present-day* lives are suffering.

These clients lament, "If only I had more time!" But the thing about time is, we only get 24 hours a day, whether we're organized or not. We'll never get more time, so learning how to better manage the time we have time is key. That's what this chapter is all about: helping our clients regain a higher quality of life *today* by learning to better manage their time.

The Three P's

When it comes to wasted time, individuals affected by CD are impacted by what I call The Three P's: perfectionism, procrastination, and paralysis. The Three P's represent internal states that lead to time-wasting behavior patterns. Perfectionism often leads to procrastination, which leads to paralysis, creating a vicious cycle.

The cycle starts with perfectionism. Many people affected by CD strive toward impossibly high standards. Having high standards is not inherently bad, but the perfectionist mindset— where things need to be *perfect*—is a trap, leading to the person feeling they can never be good enough, do the thing well enough, etc. Usually, a perfectionist engages in rigid, black-and-white thinking about their own behavior: if it's not perfect, it's not worth even trying. They take the position that only the best—that is, whatever *they* consider "the best"—will do.

Perfectionism is flawed because it does not consider any contextual factors and has little, if any, grounding in reality. Family life, career, children, money—none of these crucial life attributes are considered by the perfectionist; perfectionists believe they should be able to achieve perfection in their task no matter the circumstance. Unfortunately, even under the most ideal circumstances, "perfect" is probably not achievable at all, by anyone.

Because it's so unachievable, perfectionism is often closely paired with procrastination—the act of avoiding doing a task that needs to be accomplished. Popular media would have you believe that people procrastinate because they are lazy, but in fact, many people (including those with CD) procrastinate because they are afraid of making mistakes and not doing the task well. An online article from *Strategic Psychology* sums it up perfectly: "Perfectionists are unknowingly the masters of the art of procrastination."

Avoiding tasks can evoke feelings of self-doubt, depression, guilt, and inadequacy. To avoid these feelings, procrastinating perfectionists will start other tasks, usually more enjoyable activities that are less overwhelming. The more tasks they start, the more they leave undone, leading to feelings of overwhelm and paralysis.

To help clients escape the clutches of this paralyzing cycle, we need to do three things. First, we need to address perfectionism and procrastination. How can our clients give themselves more grace while also getting things done? This requires a mindset SHiFT®. Next, we need to help them decide *what* things they should be doing, and when. Put simply, they need help prioritizing tasks. Finally, we need to help them recognize when certain tasks are better off done by others. They need to learn to delegate.

Strive for "Good Enough"

Freeing a client from The Three P's requires changing both their mindsets and their behaviors. The individual needs to accept that perfection does not exist. No matter how hard they try, nothing they do will ever be perfect. Therefore, their goal shouldn't be perfection; it should be "good enough."

Making this change in mindset is not easy, but it is the only way they will break free of the fear that keeps them paralyzed and in a perpetual cycle of procrastination and paralysis. Procrastination "is probably the single most common hindrance to effective time management," writes Dorothy Breininger in her book *Stuff Your Face or Face Your Stuff: Lose Weight by Decluttering Your Life*. "It takes persistence to change [the habit], but you can do it."

To help your client practice striving for "good enough," encourage them to start an activity they're dreading for just five minutes and see where it goes. I tell my clients, "If, after five minutes, you don't want to do it anymore, then you can stop and do something else on your list." A lot of times, this freedom to switch tasks (as opposed to switching based on anxiety over the "hard" task) frees their mind and enables them to keep going on that first task. I've seen it firsthand! And if they do mess up the task, so what? It's an opportunity to learn and keep going.

"When I Retire"

Barbara

As you read in Chapter 6, Barbara knew her extreme quantity of belongings was weighing down her life—it's why she agreed to let me try consolidating her seven storage units. Yet as we worked together to categorize and organize the belongings in those units, I discovered that Barbara was still wasting a lot of time moving her things from one storage unit to another. She'd even take a vacation day off from work to spend time moving items around. On one day she would decide an item belonged in the unit we had dubbed "sell," and the next day she'd have moved the item back to the "keep" unit.

Fear and uncertainty were paralyzing Barbara, preventing her from sticking to her decisions. Instead, by overloading the "keep" unit, she was putting off the decision about what to do with her many belongings. It was a form of procrastinating.

"When I retire, I will have time to sort and sell my things and live a better life and focus on my hobbies," she told me.

Knowing it would take her years to sort through the remaining items individually, I questioned whether that was really how she wanted to spend her retirement. "Now is the time," I told her. "Look at your past efforts. We've come so far! If we take care of the rest of the items now, when you retire, you can immediately enjoy your hobbies." Unfortunately, Barbara had let perfectionism and its accompanying fears take hold again. She put off what could have been done today, resulting in more time lost that she could have used to pursue rest, relaxation, personal goals, and more.

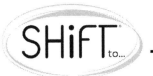

SHiFT to...

letting go of "perfect" and making "good enough" the standard.

Prioritize with the Urgent–Important Matrix

The Urgent–Important Matrix, also known as the Eisenhower Matrix, is a simple but effective framework you can use with clients to help them prioritize their to-do lists. I find that many of my clients, especially those who also have ADHD, feel an excessive sense of urgency around every task; they need to do the task *now*, no matter what it is. This results in disastrous time management, because truly important matters often get overlooked in favor of whatever the most immediate task is. The Urgent–Important Matrix helps them prioritize better.

	URGENT	NOT URGENT
IMPORTANT	**DO** *Just get it done (NOW)!*	**SCHEDULE** *I can schedule this later (YAY)!*
NOT IMPORTANT	**DELEGATE** *Take it off your plate (someone else can do it)*	**ELIMINATE** *Dump it! Bye-bye!*

The two axes on the Urgent–Important Matrix are urgency (does the task need to be done now or can it wait for later?) and importance (is it imperative this task get done, and do I need to be the one to do it?). This splits the matrix into four quadrants, each of which represents a decision about a task: Do, Schedule, Delegate, and Eliminate.

When my client indicates a task is important, we decide whether they should Do it immediately (urgent) or if they should Schedule it for later (not urgent). An urgent–important task might be picking a child up from school, while a not-urgent–important task might be laundering said child's basketball uniform for the game next weekend.

When the task is not important, it needs to be removed from the client's to-do list. Its level of urgency dictates *how* the item gets removed. If the task is not urgent and not important, it can be Eliminated entirely. These are tasks like finishing reading a magazine or writing an Amazon purchase review. If there's literally nothing else on the client's to-do list, then I tell them they're welcome to perform these tasks . . . but an empty to-do list is rarer than you might think!

Finally, if the task is not important—or, namely, not important for the client themselves to do—but it is urgent, it's time to Delegate.

Delegate Tasks You Don't Want to Do

In today's society, particularly in the United States, being self-sufficient is seen as important, bordering on essential. We want to come across as competent, and that often means avoiding asking for help. Yet we all need help sometimes, and whether we have CD or not, few of us ask as often as we should.

For individuals with CD, asking for help—which I am going to call "delegating"—is an essential way to get tasks off their plate and free up time to focus on things they enjoy and are good at. For example, Skylar was an excellent landscape architect. However, she did not have the organizational skills to run a business and would have been better off if she'd delegated all the administration work to a trusted (and trustworthy!) business partner or manager.

When I'm working with clients, I tell them, "If there are tasks you don't like or don't want to do, delegate them! Let someone else with experience handle work you don't like doing or don't know how to do." For instance, if they don't like mowing grass or shoveling snow, I find them a landscaper or a local neighborhood kid eager to make a few bucks.

Another example is taxes: if a client doesn't know how to do them and doesn't want to learn, I help them find an accountant. For these types of tasks that are difficult, hard to learn, *and* very important, delegating not only frees up my clients' time but it also gives them peace of mind. They can trust that the task is being done by an expert and will be done correctly the first time.

Thought Box

"Asking for help is a strength. What do you need help with, and whom can you ask for help?"

Creating a Daily Routine

It's important to work with clients on their mindsets and behaviors, but to make space for this work, clients need routine. And, almost without exception, routine is something people affected by CD do not have—at least until they work with a professional organizer!

Creating a general, flexible daily schedule is one of the very first things I do with clients because it frees up so much mental space. Predictable routines help establish a foundation for each day to go as smoothly as possible. They also help make chores easier, because if it's part of the routine, the decision to do the chore and any stress that might accompany that decision (Should I do this? Should I do this *now*? If I wait until later, what if I forget?) is eliminated. For activities like tidying the living room, paying the utility bill, and scheduling doctor's appointments, having a routine can help ensure that necessary activities get done when they need to be done. Then, when the errands and chores are finished, the client can spend their (free!) time doing things they're excited to do.

Building the Routine

Daily routines don't need to be complicated, and they don't need to become lengthy task lists. The two most important things to identify when building a routine are what tasks *must* be done and what activities the client really *wants* to do. For instance, tasks that must be part of an evening routine are:

- Cook and eat dinner
- Put dishes in the dishwasher
- Sleep

But dinner and dishes won't take up the whole night! Therefore, how does your client want to wind down the day? Curl up and read a book? Watch sports? Do a puzzle? Chat on the phone with a friend?

Once the dishes are loaded and the dishwasher is running, that's when they can take time to themselves. A full (yet simple) evening routine might look like this:

- Cook and eat dinner
- Put dishes in the dishwasher
- *Watch one episode of a television show OR tackle a small decluttering project*
- *Take a relaxing shower*
- *Read for 20 minutes*
- Sleep

Here's an example of a full daily schedule I created for one of my ADHD clients. It was crafted around my client's unique life demands. She posted it in her bathroom, home office, and kitchen, and even made a miniature copy to store in her car!

To create a schedule like this with a client, here are some examples of the questions I review with them:

What is the single most important thing you need to accomplish each day?

This is the activity we slot into the schedule first, and then we work around it. In the example schedule, the client's most important task was Bible study, which she called Morning Revival.

What time of the day do you feel most productive?

Whenever possible, we'll try to schedule the client's most important and urgent tasks during their most productive time of the day. In the example schedule, the client felt most productive in the morning, so that's when we scheduled her Bible study. It's also why we made time for her to reply to urgent emails before breakfast—that's when she feels her sharpest!

Is there anything you can delegate or delete from your daily schedule?

This is often a difficult question for clients to answer, so I repeat it at various intervals throughout our time together. Sometimes, it takes the client a while to experiment with daily schedules and recognize tasks they really don't need to be doing themselves, or at all. In the example schedule, the client realized that she didn't need to be the one to always pick up her children from school. As a result, she coordinated with other parents to share school pickup, which enabled her to get more done at work on those days.

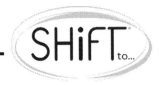

SHiFT to...

creating your ideal daily routine.

After looking at the example schedule, what would your ideal day look like?

1. Mentally list your ideal daily routine

2. Write down a flexible schedule

3. Identify the most unpredictable tasks

4. Revise the schedule

Everyone is different, so take your time creating and revising a routine that aligns with your needs. And remember: your routine can be as detailed as you like, but it always needs to remain flexible!

Building in Buffer Time

One of the most difficult parts of building a daily routine with a client is persuading them to build in buffer time. "How can I allow for more time when I already don't have enough?" they'll ask. This often leads to negotiation and numerous revisions, when they discover that thirty minutes is not, in fact, enough time to get ready for work in the morning (never mind if they get a surprise phone call, their dog has an accident, or they simply get distracted looking at social media on their phone). It can demand patience, but over time, I'm able to show them that they need to leave some room to breathe between tasks— "wiggle room" for when the unknown happens.

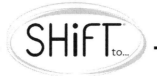

SHiFT to...

acknowledging the extra time needed to complete a task and planning for it in the future.

Writing It Down

I find it's essential to have the *client* write down the routine they develop for their day. Sure, I could draft it up and give them a copy, but there's something about them writing it down (or typing it) that gives the person an added feeling of ownership and accountability. It also helps them feel more in control when they realize they need to make a change.

There are plenty of spiral-bound planners and colorful pens at the ready if your client prefers an analog format. If they are more comfortable going digital, there are many digital software programs, like Google Calendar and iCal, and smartphone/tablet apps, like Trello and Evernote, that will do the job. Then, using the planner, program, or app, you can help your client break down their big goals into bite-sized, achievable tasks they can schedule and tackle each day.

The key to making a daily routine work is sticking to a system. Practice is essential! Even the "best," most sophisticated time management system will not work if the individual does not use it regularly and systematically. In the beginning, this will likely take a lot of reminding and encouraging on your part. It can be a long process to find what works, because each system requires a real effort to test, and sometimes the best solution is a combination of many systems. However, once the client has a system that works, they'll be amazed at how much more time they have to do things like socialize, practice self-care, and, of course, declutter! And when they realize it's the routine that's freeing up this time, they'll be all the more motivated to stick to it.

One Final Note on Routines

So far, I've emphasized the importance of building a routine and sticking to it. However, I want to add one word of caution.

There's a reason I addressed The Three P's first in this chapter: individuals affected by CD easily fall prey to perfectionism, and this extends to their daily routine. Without constant reassurance and reminders from you that this routine is a *guide*, clients can start to treat it as a hard-and-fast template they must follow at all times. When this mindset takes hold, one little deviation—which they'll see as a "failure"—can be enough to send them into a tailspin.

Personally, I find myself regularly repeating the phrase "life happens." If a client needs to spend a little more time on an activity one day, I reassure them that it's OK; it just means they'll spend a little less time on something else. If readjusting their schedule doesn't work, they can skip an activity or push it to tomorrow. This is normal! Humans are not robots, and life is unpredictable. The purpose of a routine is to provide structure— but *routines should be flexible.*

Managing "Things" That Waste Time

Even with The Three P's under control and a routine in place, individuals with CD lose precious time in one more significant way: trying to manage their "things." By "things," I mean their belongings—the many possessions filling their apartment, condo, house, and even storage units. These things are stealing their time.

So far, we've covered how a surplus of belongings can hurt our clients' social lives, their health, their sense of "I am deserving," and their finances. When it comes to time, too much "stuff" creates problems in two key ways. First, clients needlessly waste time physically looking for lost items. Second, they lose time mentally deliberating over what to do with items they feel uncertain about. Finally, just like most of us living in modern society, they lose time to items that are designed to be distracting.

Use Learning Style to Stop Losing Things

One of the biggest time sucks for individuals with CD is searching for misplaced items. People who also have ADHD particularly suffer from this issue because they not only have clutter that easily subsumes items, but they often get distracted when putting an item away and wind up setting it down somewhere else entirely, with no recollection of where that "somewhere else" was.

Decluttering helps to alleviate the issue of "losing things," of course, but I've found that reducing clutter alone doesn't give back clients nearly enough time—they still misplace important belongings and waste time hunting them down. Therefore, rather than *only* trying to create successful organization systems, I've also devised strategies to help shortcut the hunt for missing items.

The most effective strategy for a particular client is the one that best matches that client's learning style. In Denslow Brown's *The Processing Modalities Guide: Identify and Use Specific Strengths for Better Functioning*, she pinpoints several specific ways people process information and interact with their surroundings. Ultimately, she whittles them down to three sense-based learning styles: visual, auditory, and tactile. I use these categories to provide "find-it" strategies to my clients.

For example, people affected by CD often spend a lot of time searching for their car keys—often frantically, when the pressure is on to get to an appointment on time. For visual and tactile learners, I've adopted Brown's suggestion of attaching a big, bright pom-pom to the end of their keychain; the pom-pom makes the keys easier to see on a counter, and it's easy to feel and grab inside a purse. An auditory learner, on the other hand, could attach a Bluetooth tracking device like a Tile or an Apple AirTag to the keychain. This device pairs with a mobile phone, so when the person wants to find their keys, they can use their phone to trigger the Tile/AirTag, which emits a sound and makes the keys more easily discoverable.

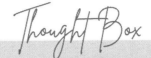

Thought Box

How do you learn best? Do you identify as a . . .

- **Visual learner**—watching a video or live person demonstrating task

- **Auditory learner**—listening to the person explain the task

- **Tactile learner**—going in and doing the task yourself

How can you use this style of learning to keep track of important items like your keys, wallet, and phone?

Paring Down "Someday" Items

While important items take up time when they're lost (and need to be found), unimportant items can take up just as much time. They do this when they're left in the limbo known as "someday."

"Someday" is perhaps the word I hear most often out of my clients' mouths: "Someday I'll know what to do with this," or "I might need this someday." The irony is that "someday" never comes, and all the "someday" items accumulate into more and more "someday" clutter, leading to discouragement and even hopelessness. Indecision can be paralyzing!

To mitigate this issue, I create a Someday Box. As we go through their belongings, any item to which they respond "I don't know" gets put into the Someday Box. For example:

Me: "Do you want to keep this belt?"

Client: "I don't know."

The belt goes into the Someday Box.

When the box is full, we label it with the current date and then agree upon a future date. If the client hasn't opened the Someday Box or used any of its contents by that later date, the box and its contents are donated or thrown away. This method helps clients escape the trap of "someday" turning into "never."

Ultimately, the Someday Box is an exercise in learning to let go. By agreeing to a timeline for (potentially) getting rid of items, the client is taking a tiny, successful step toward letting go. This method works because instead of demanding the client make a decision and release the items on the spot, it creates a delay, which allows the individual to process their feelings and come around to being okay with letting go. Through this process, they gradually learn to live lighter and freer of so many things—and when they're free of burdensome possessions, they discover more time to devote to the activities and people they love.

Setting Limits on Distracting Items

The final category of items that are stealing our clients' time is one familiar to all of us: items that are designed to be distracting. Who hasn't intended to start making breakfast only to look up from a phone screen twenty minutes later? Even a "short" break from work can quickly turn into a lost hour or more if we aren't mindful of the time passing while we're on our phone or browsing the internet. During an organizing session, one of my clients remarked, "If you weren't here, I'd be playing games on my phone." I wasn't surprised.

Many people—our clients included—use digital entertainment as a form of escape from reality and responsibility. Phones, computers, tablets, and televisions are the easiest means of escape. The apps, programs, games, and shows they contain are designed to elicit unpredictable hits of feel-good hormones, which makes them addictive, and it works.

Don—who, as you may recall from Chapter 5, eventually succumbed to substance addictions—had an incredibly hard time contending with electronic distractions. He loved his computer, TV, and cell phone—really any digital device, but especially his computer. He spent hours and hours changing his online orders, looking at his stocks, and reading the latest political news. Before he knew it, he was hopping from one internet rabbit hole to another. When he realized how much time he was wasting, he would tell me, "I just need to lie down!" Later, I would discover that he was up almost the whole night on his computer, even taking methamphetamine to keep going. His was one of the worst distraction addictions I've encountered.

Not all clients will be as affected by distracting devices, but those with ADHD are especially prone wasting large amounts of time on devices designed to steal their attention. To help them manage these types of distractions, set some healthy boundaries to limit screen time. Examples include:

- Turning off the television when they're not actively watching a program
- Shutting down the computer a few times each day
- Turning off their phone or putting it on airplane mode during designated times of the day
- Placing their phone in another room when working, eating meals, or sleeping
- Downloading an app that limits their phone time and/or time spent on specific apps
- Deleting social media apps

Decreasing Distractions
Skylar

When I worked with Skylar, I quickly realized that distractibility was a big part of her time management issues. Every morning, almost as soon as she greeted me, the phone would ring, employees would enter her office to ask questions, and clients and vendors would be vying for her attention both digitally and in person. Instead of directing calls to voicemail or asking the employee to come back at a better time, she answered the phone impulsively and immediately attended to whoever had just come in the door. After each interruption, we had to review where we had left off in our organizing session to get back on track.

After a few sessions, it was apparent that Skylar and I had gotten little accomplished because she was constantly spinning from one distraction to another. I never want to waste a client's time (or my own), so I suggested scheduling our next session during a different part of her workday in order to make the most of our time together. After some trial and error, I realized that the end of Skylar's workday was the best time to work with her, because she received fewer phone calls and had fewer client and employee interactions. During these hours, she could focus more on our organizing tasks: sorting papers, creating filing systems, and disposing of unnecessary materials.

Sometimes, as in Skylar's case, it's not possible to entirely eliminate distractions during your organizing session. In these instances, use some creativity to work within the parameters you have. Maybe changing the time of day you work with someone can make a difference. Maybe moving to a less distracting room or finding childcare for the hours when you're organizing will help. Part of our job is not just helping clients free up time in their own schedules but helping them make the most of the time they're spending with us.

Conclusion

Time is a finite asset; we can never get more of it, so we must use what we have as well as we can. Therefore, as organizers, we need to impress this message on our clients: *Your time is precious. How you choose to spend it reflects what matters most to you.*

Perfection, procrastination, and paralysis are all time-stealers, as are disorganization and distraction. To help individuals with CD take back stolen time, we can't just repeat the adage "use your time wisely;" we must work with them to put structures like daily routines and item-finding strategies in place. When they can successfully manage their time, our clients will find renewed freedom to decide how direct their energy, attention, and focus and how to ultimately fill and shape their lives. There's no better gift we can give them than that.

How did Barbara and Skylar use the "T" in SHiFT® to learn how to live a full, deserving life?

Barbara

- Inventoried her belongings using the app Airtable to identify "sell" and "keep" categories
- Began retirement activities sooner, spending more time *today* on what matters to her rather than waiting for "someday"

Skylar

- Adopted "first things first" as her new mantra
- Rerouted her calls to voicemail during times she was busy and scheduled her outgoing calls to the afternoon
- Installed a standard business operating procedure to streamline invoicing and save the time she had been spending manually looking up who hadn't yet paid for services

Think, Write...Deserve

1. Do you live in the past, present, or future? What's most comforting about living in the present? What is uncomfortable about it?

2. Describe the life you want to live. How does a daily routine facilitate that life?

3. How much time do you spend looking for misplaced items? If you could get back your lost time, how would things be different?

4. When you think about your legacy and estate planning, what steps are you taking now so your family does not have to deal with your boxes of "someday" items?

5. If you had more time to focus on yourself, how would you spend it?

Chapter 8

SHiFT®ing

SHiFT®

"We will take risks, try new things, and learn as we go."

—unknown

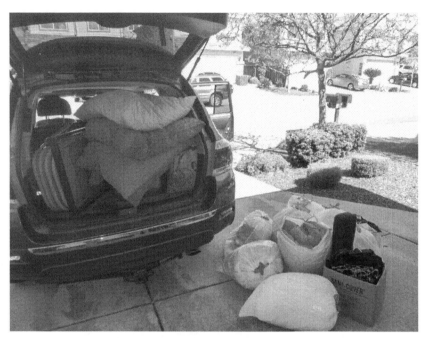

Photo credit: Connie Anderson

Unused items, on their way to be donated so someone else can benefit.

You have reached the final chapter of *Making the SHiFT*®. Bravo! I applaud you for stepping outside the confines of traditional organizing. Just by picking up this book, you recognize that working with clients affected by CD requires unique tools and techniques and that showroom-ready homes aren't the only signs of success. You also recognize the transformational power of organizing.

In the wise words of Julie Morgenstern, an internationally renowned expert and best-selling author on time management, productivity, and organizing: "When we're organized, our homes, offices, and schedules reflect and encourage who we are, what we want, and where we're going." This is the sentiment upon which the SHiFT® Method is built. For those with CD, being organized is deeply tied to that person's self-worth. The relationship is bidirectional, which is why I believe that organizers must address both the tidiness and livability of our clients' home environments *and* their self-beliefs in tandem. After reading the preceding seven chapters, it's my sincere hope that you have come to believe this, too.

SHiFT®, in Short

To create lasting change for our clients who are affected by CD, we can't just tidy their homes—we must address the full spectrum of their needs. These needs span five broad categories:

Social - Relationships and human connections that are authentic and meaningful.

Health - A physically healthy body and clean, safe home.

i am deserving - A sense of self-worth and feeling deserving of a good life.

Finances - Knowledge of money and using it to have experiences that matter.

Time - Control over one's own time and schedule to make room for fun, meaningful activities.

Every one of these categories feeds into the others, which is why we, as organizers, must help our clients address them all. Not all at once, of course; it's up to us to find the area where we can make the most significant inroads and build from there. Once the client sees progress, the trust we've begun to build will strengthen and they'll start to feel something that is integral for the SHiFT® Method to work: hope. Because with hope comes motivation and, eventually—with our help—real change.

Hank's SHiFT®

As you may have deduced, Hank's story is one of my favorite client stories to tell. When I met Hank, his daughter wouldn't even bring his granddaughter to visit him—Hank's house was that bad. Hank himself was no better; he was lonely and depressed, and his own mental and physical health were reflected in the hoarded, crumbling house around him. His CD was absolutely debilitating.

Yet Hank had hope. If he didn't, I wouldn't have been able to help him. This is the reality of working with individuals affected by CD: some individuals won't accept help because they have internalized their hopelessness. Yet others, deep inside, still believe change is possible and are ready to work toward living a deserving life—they just need help. Hank was one of these people. With patience, persistence, hard work, and some professional help from me, he transformed his home and himself.

Of course, Hank's story doesn't end with his home renovation. As Hank transitioned back into his "new" home, he had to adjust to many new things. He had to learn how to adjust the thermostat that controlled his new central heating and air conditioning. His electricity bill had slightly increased—in his case, a good problem to have, but it was something else he had to adjust to. Hank had to learn how to use the new dishwasher he'd bought, and he had to learn to trust the housekeeper I hired to come and clean on a regular basis. These were all challenging hurdles for Hank, but he worked to overcome them because he knows he is worth it.

What is so beautiful about Hank's progress is that he no longer feels trapped by old thought and behavior patterns. He knows he deserves better and has applied the SHiFT® Method to remove the unfulfilling limits of his old life. The work to live a deserving life is ongoing, but as Hank and many other clients have realized: they're worth it.

The Professional Organizing Landscape

The SHiFT® Method is part of a broader movement in professional organizing aimed at helping individuals affected by CD. New research and educational opportunities are emerging every day, which I am hopeful will make professional assistance for people affected by CD even more effective . . . and more readily available.

Thus far, I've described SHiFT® as a hands-on method. Yet sometimes, for health, scheduling, or other reasons, you cannot take your hands to your clients. This doesn't mean you can't be effective; after all, there are chronically disorganized individuals in need everywhere. And as COVID-19 taught us, many of our jobs can be done virtually—including professional organizing.

Virtual organizing is a good solution for clients who are not yet ready to invite a stranger into their homes, as well as for organizers with physical limitations and/or who want to reach a client base beyond their geographic confines. When I talk to clients, I'll often help them think through whether they would prefer virtual or in-person organizing services by using the following questions:

Should I Try Virtual Organizing?

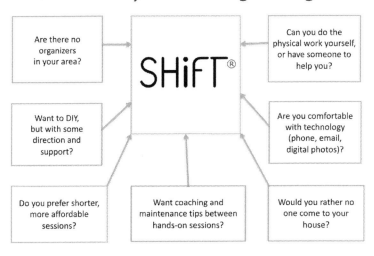

Image credit: Hazel Thornton

On the other hand, if you as a professional organizer are thinking about trying virtual organizing, here are some questions to ask before you commit:

- Are there clients you'd like to serve but whom you cannot physically reach?
- Are you willing to charge lower rates than you would for in-person organizing?
- Without you there, are your prospective clients physically able to do the organizing work?
- Will your clients be comfortable with technology (phone, email, digital photos)?

The SHiFT® Method is easily adaptable to virtual organizing so long as the answers to those last two questions are "yes." Much of the way you relate to your clients and the topics you work on will remain the same; the major difference is that building trust can take longer but is even more crucial because you will need greater levels of transparency, vulnerability, and communication from your clients in order to make progress. When you're not there in person, you can only see what they show you and must believe what they tell you. It's a different sort of challenge than organizing right alongside them, but it's no less worthy.

SHiFT® Success

The greatest privilege as a professional organizer is to watch as the SHiFT® that happens inside and outside of my client's livable spaces transforms their lives. It is why I have endeavored to share this transformative method with you through this book: so you, too, can bring out the best in your clients and witness these life-changing transformations.

Here is some of the feedback you have to look forward to when you start implementing the SHiFT® Method:

"I don't have the words to express how much you have helped me to get through the chaos in my life that has stalled me for so many years. Thank you from the bottom of my heart." - **Gretchen**

"The answer to my prayer. Actually, they go above and beyond that. They lit a fire within me. They offer steadfast support, guidance, and encouragement along your journey. As a result, I feel more in control, less overwhelmed by clutter, and more proactive. It's like getting out of jail from the chaos and finally feeling free!" - **Barbara**

"[Learning to live a deserving life] has been a godsend, and it is a pleasure to work with them! After too many years of 'collecting' and hoarding behavior, I am now challenged with dealing with the result. I often become overwhelmed, lose motivation, and am unable to move forward. Jen knows just how to tackle whatever the challenge might be and knows right where to start and dig in headfirst. Throughout the process, she is encouraging, supportive, and knows just the right amount of nudging to keep things moving toward your goal without making you feel like you have lost control of the process. We have only gone a short way on the long path ahead, but I know with her expertise, energy, and support, I am going to be successful in reaching my goal of having a well-appointed, uncluttered environment." - **Hank**

It's Time to Go Forth

At last, it's time to put what you've learned into practice. Are you excited? Do you feel ready?

It's OK if you're nervous about putting the SHiFT® Method into practice. Especially if you're new to professional organizing or have been using the same tactics for years or even decades, trepidation is to be expected! The best thing to do is to start small. Begin by asking your clients a simple set of questions, which I've adapted from Denslow Brown's *Coach Approach for Organizers* training course:

- What are you seeing, hearing, or feeling?
- What is a win?
- What's getting in the way?
- What's hard, tough, or scary?
- What lifestyle changes have you achieved that are rewarding?
- What lifestyle changes do you hope to achieve?

These questions get at the heart of who your clients are and what they want. Their answers will help you determine whether Social, Health, "i am deserving," Finances, or Time is the best place to start.

Of course, as you make progress together, your clients will certainly have questions—and I suspect you will, too. That's why I've developed the SHiFT® Training Academy. This six-week course delves even deeper into the fundamentals of organizing with the SHiFT® Method and prepares you to become a certified SHiFT® specialist.

To learn more, visit http://livablespaces.net.

Let's SHiFT® lives!

ACKNOWLEDGMENTS

To Judith Kolberg: Thank you for your mentorship, guidance, and support over my many years of organizing. You offered me encouragement in my earliest days of writing, before I ever believed finishing an entire book would be possible. Without you and the foundation of knowledge you have provided, *Making the SHiFT®* would not exist.

To my contributor, Connie Anderson: This book is richer for the stories and input you have provided. Thank you so much for the time and effort you put into reading various drafts of this manuscript. As we both came to recognize, writing is one thing, but revision is quite another!

To my husband, Marc; my kids, Sophie and Cooper; and my stepfather, Brad Wiley: While I spent countless hours away from you to write this book and then revise it, you were more patient and supportive than I could ever have expected. Thank you from the bottom of my heart.

To my clients: The trust you placed in me as you invited me into your homes and your lives is what made the SHiFT® Method possible. Thank you for your vulnerability and for helping to share the power of organizing with others seeking to live deserving lives. You are my inspiration every day.

Finally, to all of my past, present, and future fellow organizers: Thank you for taking up this profession. Together, we are making a difference in the lives of people affected by CD. Together, we are SHiFT®ing minds and transforming lives to make the world a better place.

NOTES

Chapter 1: Identifying Chronic Disorganization

1. American Psychiatric Association. (2013). *Diagnostic and statistical manual of mental disorders* (5th ed.). https://doi.org/10.1176/appi.books.9780890425596

Chapter 2: Introducing the SHiFT® Method

1. Lagacé, M. (n.d.). *100 Change Quotes that Will Fuel Your Growth.* https://wisdomquotes.com/change-quotes/

2. Quintana, D., & Beattie, J. S. (2020). *Filled up and overflowing: What to do when life events, chronic disorganization, or hoarding go overboard.* Release Repurpose Reorganize LLC.

3. Varness, K. (Ed.). (2012). *The ICD guide to challenging disorganization: For professional organizers.* Institute for Challenging Disorganization.

4. Institute for Challenging Disorganization. (n.d.). *The ICD® Clutter–Hoarding Scale®.* https://www.challengingdisorganization.org/clutter-hoarding-scale-

Chapter 3: "S" Is for Social

1. Tate, N. (2018, May 4). Loneliness rivals obesity, smoking as health risk. *WebMD.* https://www.webmd.com/balance/news/20180504/loneliness-rivals-obesity-smoking-as-health-risk

2. O'Sullivan, R., Burns, A. Leavey, G., Leroi, I, Burholt, V., Luben, J., Holt-Lunstad, J., Victor, C., Lawlor, B., Vilar-Compte, M., Perissinotto, C. M., Tully, M. A., Sullivan, M. P., Rosato, M., Power, J. M., Tiilikaninen, E., & Prohaska, T. R. (2021). Impact of COVID-19 pandemic on loneliness and social isolation: A multi-country study. *International Journal of Environmental Research on Public Health, 18*(19), 9982. https://doi.org/10.3390/ijerph18199982

3. Kessler, R. C., Adler, L., Barkley, R., Biederman, J., Conners, K., Demler, O., Faraone, S. V., Greenhill, L. L., Howes, M. J., Secnik, K., Spencer, T. Ustun, B., Walters, E. E., and Zaslavsky, A. M. (2006). The prevalence and correlates of adult ADHD in the United States: Results from the National Comorbidity Survey replication. *The American Journal of Psychiatry, 163*(4), 716–723. https://doi.org/10.1176/appi.ajp.163.4.716

4. Psychology Today. (n.d.). *Polyamory.* https://www.psychologytoday.com/us/basics/polyamory

5. Noe Pagán, C. (2015). ADHD and risky behavior in adults. *WebMD.* https://www.webmd.com/add-adhd/guide/adhd-dangerous-risky-behavior

6. Astryan, K. (2015). 4 disorders that may thrive on loneliness. *Psychology Today.* https://www.psychologytoday.com/us/blog/the-art-closeness/201507/4-disorders-may-thrive-loneliness

7. Cacioppo, J., & Patrick, W., (2008). *Loneliness: Human nature and the need for social connection.* W. W. Norton & Company.

8. Lehmiller, J. J. (2019). Do people with ADHD have a harder time with monogamy? *Psychology Today.* https://www. psychologytoday.com/us/blog/the-myths-sex/201910/do-people-adhd-have-harder-time-monogamy

Chapter 4: "H" Is for Health

1. MedicalNewsToday. (2020, April 19). *What is good health?* https://www.medicalnewstoday. com/articles/150999what_is_health

2. Healthline. (2021, December 14). *Top 10 benefits of exercise.* https://www.healthline.com/ nutrition/10-benefits-of-exercise

3. Varness, K. (Ed.). (2012). *The ICD guide to challenging disorganization: For professional organizers.* Institute for Challenging Disorganization.

Chapter 5: "i" Is for I Am Deserving

1. Yesko, J. (2021). *I'm right here: 10 ways to get help for hoarding and chronic disorganization.* Academy Press.

2. International OCD Foundation. (n.d.). https:// www.iocdf.org/

Chapter 6: "F" Is for Financial

1. Institute for Challenging Disorganization. (n.d.). *Common Characteristics of Individuals Affected by Chronic Disorganization.* https://www.challengingdisorganization. org/assets/ICDPublications/FactSheets/ ICD%20fs003%20Characteristics%20of%20 Individuals%20Affected%20by%20Chronic%20 Disorganization%202019.pdf

2. Psychology Today. (n.d.). *The Call of the Mall.* https://www.psychologytoday.com/us/ articles/199501/the-call-the-mall

Chapter 7: "T" Is for Time

1. Strategic Psychology. (n.d.). *Procrastination: Your perfectionism may be the problem.* https:// strategicpsychology.com.au/procrastination-your-perfectionism-may-be-the-problem/

2. Ferrari, J. R. (2010). *Still procrastinating. The no-regrets guide to getting it done.* John Wiley and Sons.

3. Psychology Today. (n.d.). *Procrastination.* https://www.psychologytoday.com/us/basics/ procrastination

4. Breininger, D. (2013). *Stuff Your Face or Face Your Stuff: Lose Weight by Decluttering Your Life.* Health Communications, Inc.

5. Productfolio. (n.d.). Eisenhower Matrix (Urgent vs. Important). https://productfolio.com/ eisenhower-matrix/

6. Brown, D. (2010). *The processing modalities guide: Identify and use specific strengths for better functioning*. **Hickory Guild Press.**

7. Tuckman, A. (2009). *More attention, less deficit: Success strategies for adults with ADHD.* **Specialty Press.**

Chapter 8: SHiFT®ing

1. Brown, D. (2016). *The coach approach for organizers: Powerful questions* **[handout]**.

APPENDICES

Appendix A

The ICD® Factors Associated with Disorganization

Disorganization can be caused by many factors. Determining the cause(s) of one's disorganization and finding solutions to overcoming it can be aided with the assistance of a professional organizer, particularly one trained in dealing with CD.

The chart on the next page offers limited examples within each category and should not be considered all-inclusive.

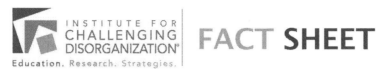

INSTITUTE FOR
CHALLENGING
DISORGANIZATION®
Education. Research. Strategies.

FACT SHEET

Factors Associated with Disorganization

Disorganization can be caused by many factors. Determining the cause(s) of one's disorganization and finding solutions to overcoming it can be aided with the assistance of a professional organizer, particularly one trained in dealing with chronic disorganization.

BRAIN-BASED CONDITIONS	BELIEFS ABOUT SELF / POSSESSIONS	SITUATIONAL FACTORS

The following chart offers limited examples within each category and should not be considered all-inclusive.

Neurologically-Based Conditions	Learning Styles or Modalities	Perfectionism
• Attention Deficit Hyperactivity Disorder (ADHD) • Traumatic brain injury (TBI) • Fibromyalgia • Parkinson's Disease • Multiple sclerosis (MS)	• System not well suited to the individual's learning style or modality • Visual thinker who believes "out of sight, out of mind" • Tactile sympathy • Holistic thinker	• Leaving things undone due to a fear of making a mistake • Acquiring more than is necessary to make things perfect • Spending too much time doing something in an effort to make it "perfect"
Mental Health Issues	**Information-Processing Deficits**	**Attachments to Possessions**
• Depression • Anxiety disorder • Avoidance disorder • Social anxiety disorder • Obsessive Compulsive Disorder (OCD) • Compulsive Hoarding Disorder	• Decision-making difficulty • Distractibility • Memory deficits • Categorization difficulties	• Over-attachment to objects due to: ◦ Sentimental reasons ◦ Instrumental reasons ◦ Intrinsic reasons
Addictive Tendencies	**Learning Differences**	**Beliefs and Attitudes**
• Compulsive acquisition • Infomania • Urgency addiction • Compulsive saving • Drug and/or alcohol addiction	• Dyslexia • Dyscalculia • Dysgraphia • Auditory processing disorder • Nonverbal learning disability	• False beliefs such as: I am a procrastinator; I always have been, and always will be. • Fear of making a mistake or being judged poorly by others
Aging Issues	**Emotional and/or Behavioral Patterns**	**Ineffective Beliefs about Possessions**
• Physical difficulties • Medications • Cognitive problems	• Procrastination & avoidance • Acquiring or saving objects as a result of emotional reactions	• Unrealistically valuing objects • Associating possessions with one's identity • Sense of obligation to take care of objects
Physical Challenges	**Communication Problems**	**Choices**
• Impaired mobility • Fatigue • Poor vision • Dysphasia • Sleep disorder	• Poor negotiation skills • Conflicting communication styles among family members or colleagues at work • Weak management, leadership, and delegation strategies	• Over scheduling • Too much stuff • No sense of mission • Not setting short or long-term goals • Misplaced priorities
Life Crises	**Transitions**	**Systemic Factors**
• Health emergency • Death of a loved one • Automobile accident • Job loss • Family crisis • Trauma	• One or more moves • Relocation Stress Syndrome • Birth or adoption of a child • Parents or adult children move in • Divorce or separation	• No system • Ineffective system, such as one that is overly complex or too difficult to implement
Lack of Skills	**Environmental Factors**	
• Never taught in school • Poor modeling by parents or guardians • Churning	• Poor lighting • Lack of storage space • Awkward traffic flow • Unpleasant space • House renovation	

ICD Fact Sheet – 004
By Phyllis Flood Knerr, CPO-CD®

Source: https://www.challengingdisorganization.org/assets/ICDPublications/FactSheets/ICD%20fs005%20Time%20Management%20Tips%20for%20Individuals%20or%20Households%20Affected%20by%20CD%202019.pdf

Appendix B

The ICD® Clutter–Hoarding Scale®

The Clutter–Hoarding Scale® is an assessment tool, developed by the Institute for Challenging Disorganization® (ICD®) to give professional organizers and related professionals definitive parameters related to health and safety. The scale has established five levels to indicate the degree of household clutter and/or hoarding from the perspective of a professional organizer or related professional. The levels in the scale are progressive, with Level I as the lowest and Level V the highest. ICD® considers Level III to be the pivot point between a household that might be assessed as cluttered and a household assessment that may require the deeper considerations of working in a hoarding environment.

ICD's CLUTTER–HOARDING SCALE® FIVE CATEGORIES.

Structure and Zoning
Assessment of access to entrances and exits; function of plumbing, electrical, HVAC (any aspect of heating, ventilation or air conditioning) systems and appliances; and structural integrity

Animals and Pests
Assessment of animal care and control; compliance with local animal regulations; assessment for evidence of infestations of pests (rodents, insects or other vermin)

Household Functions
Assessment of safety, functionality and accessibility of rooms for intended purposes

Health and Safety
Assessment of sanitation levels in household; household management of medications for prescribed (Rx) and/or over-the-counter (OTC) drugs

Personal Protective Equipment (PPE)
Recommendations for PPE (face masks, gloves, eye shields or clothing that protect wearer from environmental health and safety hazards); additional supplies as appropriate to observational level

SCOPE OF SCALE
PURPOSE OF SCALE: This document is to be used as an assessment/guideline tool only, specifically for use in the assessment of a home's interior, except where the outside structure affects the overall safety of the interior. Does not include sheds, unattached garages or outbuildings. It is not to be used for diagnostic purposes or for any psychological evaluation of a person or persons. ICD is not responsible for any work performed by a professional organizer or other related professional using ICD's C–HS® or C–HS® Quick Reference Guide.

ICD's CLUTTER–HOARDING SCALE® FIVE LEVELS.

Five progressive levels indicate the degree of household clutter and/or hoarding; Level I as the lowest, and Level V the highest. ICD considers Level III as the pivot point between a household that might be assessed as cluttered, and a household environment that may require the deeper considerations of working in a hoarding environment.

LEVEL I   GREEN   LOW
Household environment is considered standard. No special knowledge in working with the chronically disorganized is necessary.

LEVEL II   BLUE   GUARDED
Household environment requires professional organizers or related professionals who have additional knowledge and understanding of chronic disorganization.

LEVEL III   YELLOW   ELEVATED
Pivot point between a cluttered household environment and a potential hoarding environment. Those working with Level III household environments should have significant training in chronic disorganization and will require a community network of resources, especially mental health professionals.

LEVEL IV   ORANGE   HIGH
Household environment requires a coordinated collaborative team of service providers in addition to professional organizers and family; mental health professionals, social workers, financial counselors, pest and animal control officers, crime scene cleaners, licensed contractors and handypersons.

LEVEL V   RED   SEVERE
Professional organizers should not work alone in a Level V environment. Requires a collaborative team, potentially including family, mental health professionals, social workers, building manager, zoning, fire, and/or safety agents. Formal written agreements among the parties should be in place before proceeding.

COPYRIGHT: ©2019 The Institute for Challenging

Source: https://www.challengingdisorganization.org/assets/ICDPublications/C-HS/ICD%20C-HS%202019%20Quick%20Guide.pdf

Appendix C

Making the SHiFT® Client Discovery Form

The purpose of the following questions is to determine the impact of how chronic disorganization (CD) has affected your life, and how by making your space livable will also SHiFT® your perspective. SHiFT® is an acronym for Social, Health, "i" Am Deserving, Finance, and Time—areas that are most impacted by CD. The SHiFT® Method is an integrated method to organize and evolve organically over time. The method helps you to address organizing from all angles, allowing for a more deserving life. You'll learn new practical skills, become more self-aware, and learn new positive habits. With continued practice, you'll feel hopeful and fulfilled.

"S" SOCIAL

Tell me about your family, friends, close social circle, and support groups.

"H" HEALTH

Tell me about how CD has shown up as it relates to your physical health and the health of your home.

"i" I AM DESERVING

Tell me about how you're feeling (mental state of mind). Have you been diagnosed?

"F" FINANCES

How has CD shown up regarding your finances (late payments, collections, excessive shopping, storage units, bankruptcy)?

"T" TIME

Do you use a planner/calendar/phone app to manage your time or set goals? Are you on time to appointments and realistically estimate how long a task will take?

Appendix D

Making the SHiFT® Questionnaire

Please answer the following questions openly. (Psst, don't overthink the questions!)

Not me!	Sometimes	Not sure/Not applicable	Kinda agree	Yes, that's me!
1	2	3	4	5

"S" SOCIAL

Are you feeling lonely or depressed?

Not me!   1   2   3   4   5   Yes, that's me!

When it comes to my family and friends, they barely ever visit any more.

Not me!   1   2   3   4   5   Yes, that's me!

It's very important to me to have material possessions more than personal connections.

Not me!   1   2   3   4   5   Yes, that's me!

My pet(s) are all I need.

Not me!   1   2   3   4   5   Yes, that's me!

Do you feel overwhelmed and anxious?

Not me!   1   2   3   4   5   *Yes, that's me!*

"H" HEALTH

When it comes to eating a nutritious meal, I don't have enough counter space to make anything.

Not me!   1   2   3   4   5   *Yes, that's me!*

I don't like to cook (or I don't have time), so I get takeout or microwave!

Not me!   1   2   3   4   5   *Yes, that's me!*

I don't like to take walks or exercise, it's just not that important.

Not me!   1   2   3   4   5   *Yes, that's me!*

Our family (or I) don't eat at the dining room table because there's too much clutter on the kitchen table.

Not me!   1   2   3   4   5   *Yes, that's me!*

Our family (or I) is/am too busy, so we/I just eat wherever we/I can find a place to sit, usually in front of the TV or computer.

Not me!   1   2   3   4   5   *Yes, that's me!*

"i" I AM DESERVING

I like/love lots of stuff around me.

Not me!   1   2   3   4   5   *Yes, that's me!*

I feel safe and secure with lots of stuff around me.

Not me!   **1   2   3   4   5**   *Yes, that's me!*

I don't feel worthy or deserving of a clean, clutter-free, livable space.

Not me!   **1   2   3   4   5**   *Yes, that's me!*

Even if I wanted a more livable space, I'm so overwhelmed!

Not me!   **1   2   3   4   5**   *Yes, that's me!*

I want to live in a clutter-free space, but I'm afraid of losing my stuff, my memories.

Not me!   **1   2   3   4   5**   *Yes, that's me!*

"F" FINANCIAL

Every time I can't find something, I just buy more.

Not me!   **1   2   3   4   5**   *Yes, that's me!*

I can afford to buy whatever I want/need, so it doesn't matter if I already have multiple items.

Not me!   **1   2   3   4   5**   *Yes, that's me!*

I have a lot of debt, but I just don't think about it, it would make me so upset.

Not me!   **1   2   3   4   5**   *Yes, that's me!*

I have incurred a lot of late fees/collections, because the bills slide to the back of the table and I can't find them.

Not me!   **1   2   3   4   5**   *Yes, that's me!*

If I knew how to use "bill pay" and "go green" I probably would.

Not me!   1   2   3   4   5   Yes, that's me!

"T" TIME

I am always late to an appointment, because I can't find my keys or other items I need to take with me.

Not me!   1   2   3   4   5   Yes, that's me!

I would like to use a planner or digital calendar, but I don't know where to find the "perfect" calendar for me.

Not me!   1   2   3   4   5   Yes, that's me!

I just don't have time to keep my home livable.

Not me!   1   2   3   4   5   Yes, that's me!

I don't have time to exercise and eat healthy. It's the last thing I think about.

Not me!   1   2   3   4   5   Yes, that's me!

I have not thought about estate planning. It seems too far off in the future or uncomfortable to deal with.

Not me! **1   2   3   4   5**   *Yes, that's me!*

For the Professional Organizer

Scoring: Add up the scores from each question in each category. Sum the categories individually (Social, Health, etc.) to see which are the highest, and then collectively. For the collective score:

1–25 = Low, meaning your daily personal behavior is not too bothered by your clutter

26–50 = Elevated, meaning your daily personal behavior is slightly bothered

51–75 = Tipping point, meaning your daily personal behavior is significantly affected

76–100 = High, meaning your daily behavior is causing a great deal of stress, overwhelm, anxiety, etc.

101–125 = Severe, meaning your daily behavior is causing so much stress, overwhelm, and anxiety you feel paralyzed

For clients on the "low" end of the SHiFT® scale, the five areas of SHiFT® really don't affect their day-to-day behavior and organizational skills. The "elevated" SHiFT® score, like the "low" SHiFT® score, means they may not feel overwhelmed by their clutter and their behavior and organizational skills are not an issue. Then the "tipping point" is where they're feeling and noticing overwhelm and anxiety, and issues in the five categories of SHiFT® are magnified. When they score "high" to "severe," the impact of issues in Social, Health, "i" am deserving, Finances, and Time impact their daily life in a significant way.

The higher a client scores, the more areas in their life will feel the benefit of SHiFT®, once addressed. The lower their score, the fewer areas they will need to concentrate on. However, even if they have a lower overall score, a relatively high score in one area (for example, 20–25 in Health) can indicate where you and your client will want to direct your efforts.

Using multiple scales: Before I meet with a potential client, I typically have them complete both this SHiFT® questionnaire and the Making the SHiFT® Client Discovery Form (Appendix C). Then, when I'm assessing their home, I also use the ICD® Clutter–Hoarding Scale®. The reason is that the SHiFT® scale focuses on intangible areas of your client's life, whereas the ICD® Clutter–Hoarding Scale® was developed by the Institute for Challenging Disorganization® (ICD®) to give professional organizers and related professionals definitive parameters *related to health and safety of the client's home*. Therefore, both have a place in your initial client assessment.

Appendix E

SHiFT® Resources for Further Exploration

"S" is for Social

Associations
- Attention Deficit Disorder Association
- Anxiety and Depression Association of America
- International OCD Foundation
- International Association for Relationship Research: https://iarr.org

Books
- *S*ocial Being by Susan Fiske (2003)
- Belong: Find Your People, Create Community, and Life a more Connected Life by Radha Agrawal (2018)
- Together: The Healing Power of Human Connection in a Sometimes Lonely World by Viverk H. Murthy (2020)

Podcasts
- The Science of Happy
- Mindful Communication with host Jonathan Miller
- A Slob Comes Clean

Websites
- Edge: https://www.edge.org/response-detail/25395
- Psychology Today: https://www.psychologytoday.com/us/blog/what-would-aristotle-do/201009/you-are-social-animal
- The Conversation: https://theconversation.com/coronavirus-experts-in-evolution-explain-why-social-distancing-feels-so-unnatural-134271
- Healthline: https://www.healthline.com/health/adhd/adult-adhd-sex-lifetreatment

"H" is for Health

Associations

- Association for Better Health
- Hope and Healing Center
- American Heart Association

Books

- The Organized Kitchen: Keep Your Kitchen Clean, Organized, and Full of Good Food and Save Time, Money and Your Sanity Every Day! by Brette Sember (2011)
- Organizing your Kitchen with Sort and Succeed by Darla deMorrow (2018)

Podcasts

- US News Top 10 Nutrition Podcasts: https://health.usnews.com/health-news/blogs/eat-run/articles/2016-10-04/10-nutrition-podcasts-to-add-to-your-playlist

Websites

- Kitchen Organization Products: https://self.com/gallery/kitchen-organization-products
- Our Happy Hive: https://OurHappyHive.com

"i" is for I Am Deserving

Associations

- Choosing Therapy
- National Center for Emotional Wellness
- National Association for Self-Esteem

Books

- Own Your Self: The Surprising Path beyond Depression, Anxiety, and Fatigue to Reclaiming Your Authenticity, Vitality, and Freedom by Kelly Brogan (2019)
- Maybe You Should Talk to Someone: A Therapist, HER Therapist, and Our Lives Revealed by Lori Gottlieb (2019)
- Your Happiness Toolkit: 16 Strategies for Overcoming Depression, and Building a Joyful, Fulfilling Life by Carrie M. Wrigley (2019)

Podcasts
- Worthy
- On Purpose with Jay Shetty
- Happier with Gretchen Rubin

Websites
- Inc.com: https://www.inc.com/nicolas-cole/7-steps-to-transform-yourself-from-who-you-are-to-who-you-want-to-be.html
- My Coach Match: https://web.mycoachmatch.com/register/survey.aspx?type=client
- Dependable Divas: https://dependable-divas.com/help-for-hoarders-and-chronically-disorganized/

"F" is for Financial

Associations
- The Association of Financial Professionals
- Financial Management Association
- CNBC Make It
- Shopping Addictions, The Shulman Center
- Debt, Debtors Anonymous

Books
- Women & Money by Suze Orman (2007)
- Overspending To Buy or Not to Buy: Why We Overshop and How to Stop by April Lane Benson (2008)
- I Will Teach You To Be Rich by Ramit Sethi (2009)
- The Simple Path to Wealth by J. L. Collins (2016)

Podcasts
- So Money
- Mad Fientist
- The Balance

Websites

- Smart About Money (SAM): https://www.smartaboutmoney.org/Topics/Holidays-and-Money/Save-Money-This-Summer/Get-Organized-and-Clean-Up-Your-Finances
- You Need a Budget: https://www.youneedabudget.com
- Money Management: https://moneymanagement.org/blog/manage-your-time-and-master-your-money

"T" is for Time

Associations

- American Management Association
- Skill Path
- Learning Tree International

Books

- The 7 Habits of Highly Effective People: Powerful Lessons in Personal Change by Stephen R. Covey (1989)
- Time Warrior: How to Defeat Procrastination, People-pleasing, Self-doubt, Over-commitment, Broken Promises and Chaos by Steve Chandler (2011)

Podcasts

- Take Back Time with Penny Zenker
- Before Breakfast with Laura Vanderkam
- Ditch Busy

Websites

- SPICA: https://www.spica.com/blog/time-management-skills
- Redbooth: https://redbooth.com/hub/time-management-strategy/
- Freshbooks: https://www.freshbooks.com/hub/productivity/importance-of-time-management

GLOSSARY

Attention Deficit Hyperactivity Disorder (ADHD).
A neurodevelopmental disorder, meaning a condition that is due to differences in the development and function of the nervous system, characterized by developmentally inappropriate levels of inattention, impulsivity, and hyperactivity.

Backsliding. The term used to describe reverting to old habits at the expenses of new goals.

Chronic Disorganization (CD). A state of disorganization consisting of three conditions: persists over a long period of time, frequently undermines the quality of life, and recurs despite repeated self-help attempts, with future expectation of more disorganization.

Cleanout. A purge and reorganization of a space, room, or entire home, often performed by someone who is not living in the home.

Harm Reduction Theory. In the context of organizing, refers to taking measures to reduce potential physical dangers in a home environment.

ICD. Institute for Challenging Disorganization.

Obsessive-Compulsive Disorder (OCD). A mental health disorder that features a pattern of unwanted thoughts and fears (obsessions) that lead the person to do repetitive behaviors (compulsions). These obsessions and compulsions interfere with daily activities and cause significant distress.

Polyamory. The practice of engaging in multiple romantic (and typically sexual) relationships, with the consent of all the people involved.

Post-Traumatic Stress Disorder (PTSD). A condition of persistent mental and emotional stress occurring as a result of injury or severe psychological shock, typically involving disturbance of sleep and constant vivid recall of the experience, with dulled responses to others and to the outside world.

Stroke. A sudden disabling attack or loss of consciousness caused by an interruption in the flow of blood to the brain.

Traumatic Brain Injury (TBI). A brain injury caused by external force, such as a blow to the head, and which results in temporary or permanent symptoms including impairments in cognition, emotional and behavioral changes, headaches, dizziness, fatigue, seizures, blurred vision, loss of taste or smell, impaired coordination, and/or numbness or paralysis of an extremity.

ABOUT THE AUTHOR

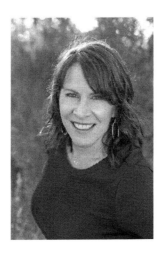

Photo credit: Lisa Westphal Photography

Jen Cazares is a Certified Professional Organizer in Chronic Disorganization®, Certified Virtual Organizing Professional™, and principal and owner of Livable Spaces®, LLC. She has spent nearly a decade working with hundreds of clients affected by hoarding disorder, attention deficit hyperactivity disorder (ADHD), post-traumatic stress disorder (PTSD), traumatic brain injury (TBI), and other factors associated with chronic disorganization. She uses her past careers, current passions, and endless empathy to make meaningful, lasting, life-changing connections with her clients. Jen lives in Concord, California, with her husband Marc; her two children, Sophie and Cooper; and their three dogs, Marley, Charlie, and Peetie.

ABOUT THE CONTRIBUTOR

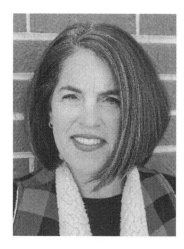

Photo credit: Jackie Doyle

Connie Anderson, Certified Professional Organizer in Chronic Disorganization®, is the owner and operator of Anderson Organizing based in Coeur d'Alene, Idaho. Her home bustles with the commotion of a cat, dogs, husband, and two sons. Born and raised in California, she regularly visits her clients to continue to provide support. During her twenty-five-year career, she remains an active networker and community builder. Her life is ever full.

Made in the USA
Columbia, SC
21 August 2023

21847553R00107